STRAP TAPING FOR SPORTS AND REHABILITATION

Anne Keil, BS, PT, DPT

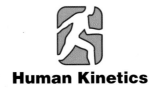

Human Kinetics

Library of Congress Cataloging-in-Publication Data

Keil, Anne, 1967-

   Strap taping for sports and rehabilitation / Anne Keil.
     p. ; cm.
   Includes bibliographical references.
   ISBN-13: 978-0-7360-9527-3 (print)
   ISBN-10: 0-7360-9527-6 (print)
   I. Title.
   [DNLM: 1. Athletic Injuries--rehabilitation. 2. Athletic Tape. 3. Braces. 4. Orthopedic
Procedures--methods. 5.
Physical Therapy Modalities. QT 261]
   617.1'027--dc23

               2011035628

ISBN-10: 0-7360-9527-6 (print)
ISBN-13: 978-0-7360-9527-3 (print)

Acquisitions Editors: Loarn D. Robertson, PhD, and Melinda Flegel; **Developmental Editor:** Kevin Matz; **Assistant Editor:** Steven Calderwood; **Copyeditor:** Patricia L. MacDonald; **Permissions Manager:** Dalene Reeder; **Graphic Designer:** Joe Buck; **Graphic Artist:** Kathleen Boudreau-Fuoss; **Cover Designer:** Keith Blomberg; **DVD Face Designer:** Susan Allen; **Photographer (cover):** Neil Bernstein; **Photographers (interior):** Neil Bernstein and Jason Allen; **Visual Production Assistants:** Joyce Brumfield and Amy Rose; **Photo Production Manager:** Jason Allen; **Art Manager:** Kelly Hendren; **Associate Art Manager:** Alan L. Wilborn; **Illustrations:** Primal Pictures, Ltd., unless otherwise noted; **Printer:** Versa Press

Printed in the United States of America   10   9   8   7   6   5   4   3   2   1

Human Kinetics
Website: www.HumanKinetics.com

United States: Human Kinetics
P.O. Box 5076
Champaign, IL 61825-5076
800-747-4457
e-mail: humank@hkusa.com

Canada: Human Kinetics
475 Devonshire Road Unit 100
Windsor, ON N8Y 2L5
800-465-7301 (in Canada only)
e-mail: info@hkcanada.com

Europe: Human Kinetics
107 Bradford Road
Stanningley
Leeds LS28 6AT, United Kingdom
+44 (0) 113 255 5665
e-mail: hk@hkeurope.com

Australia: Human Kinetics
57A Price Avenue
Lower Mitcham, South Australia 5062
08 8372 0999
e-mail: info@hkaustralia.com

New Zealand: Human Kinetics
P.O. Box 80
Torrens Park, South Australia 5062
0800 222 062
e-mail: info@hknewzealand.com

E5179

CONTENTS

PREFACE

Taping is a therapeutic bracing intervention that helps support or control joint mobility during activity. It is a low-cost procedure that can replace the need for expensive and cumbersome custom and off-the-shelf bracing, and most anyone can apply strapping tape effectively with proper instruction.

My first introduction to taping was during a seminar in my first year as a physical therapist in 1991. The seminar was taught by a physical therapist who had spent years as an athlete and athletic trainer. It opened my eyes to the amazing effect a little roll of tape can have on the human body.

For as long as I can remember, I have had problems sitting for long periods of time on bleachers, stools, and other objects that lack back support because my back and neck felt very uncomfortable. As part of that seminar, we sat up straight in proper neutral posture and then taped each other's backs, covering all the skin from the top of the shoulder blades down to the waistline with athletic tape. We wore the tape on our backs for the rest of the day as we were sitting on the treatment tables. I was amazed that my back and neck weren't tired at all—it felt as if my back was supported, so my muscles didn't have to work as hard.

I decided to try these techniques in the physical therapy clinic, but I didn't have athletic tape. So, over the years I experimented with different techniques using Leukotape (hereafter referred to as strapping tape) and Cover-Roll (skin-protectant underwrap tape) to reproduce what I had learned in the seminar. In the pages that follow, some of these orthopedic taping techniques are demonstrated along with some common techniques developed and used by Jenny McConnell, PT, and Brian Mulligan, PT, among others. I have seen amazing results after applying these techniques and have taught them to many therapists, patients, and family members. Many of these techniques can also be used or modified for use with the neurological and pediatric populations.

This text and DVD are an excellent teaching reference for physical therapists (PTs), physical therapist assistants (PTAs), occupational therapists (OTs), occupational therapy assistants (COTAs), athletic trainers (ATCs), and students and faculty in these fields. Any health care professional or layperson (e.g., coach, athlete) will also benefit from this material, when there has been a proper assessment of an injury and the taping application is under the direction of a trained professional. The text combines both physical therapy taping techniques and modified athletic training taping techniques used on all body areas into one easy-to-use reference guide, and each taping technique is also demonstrated on the accompanying DVD. Look for the **DVD** near each technique included on the DVD. Knowledge of anatomy and biomechanics is helpful for the reader to apply these techniques correctly. Some vocabulary will be common knowledge to physical therapists and other health professionals, although perhaps not to the layperson or beginning student.

In addition to an explanation of taping techniques, the text includes pictures of useful surface anatomical references and landmarks, functional range of motion reviews, current evidence supporting the efficacy of taping, screenings used to determine the appropriate taping technique to apply, braces that can simulate or be a substitute for taping if need be, and sequential photos demonstrating the techniques. The rationale used for taping for various injuries and diagnoses in each chapter as well as case studies to illustrate patient and therapist experiences in which the taping was effective are also provided.

Chapter 1 describes the types of tape available and currently used for taping, theories about why taping is effective, taping precautions, supplies, and guidelines for taping application. Chapter 2 addresses taping techniques for the ankle and foot, orthotics use, and footwear. Chapter 3 explains taping techniques for the knee and when heel lifts are appropriate to consider for treatment. Chapter 4 outlines taping techniques for the cervical, thoracic, and lumbo-pelvic area. Chapter 5 discusses techniques for the shoulder and scapula. Chapter 6 addresses the elbow, wrist, and hand.

Let's start taping!

ACKNOWLEDGMENTS

Ongoing thanks to friends and family who inspire me.

A big thank you to John Hermanstorfer of Patterson Medical, Denver, for donating all the taping supplies and some of the brace examples for this book. And to University of Colorado Hospital Outpatient Rehabilitation Clinics for use of other brace examples, to Superfeet for donating a product sample, and to Sole Supports, Inc. for the wonderful orthotic that enables me to hike nonstop.

Thanks to the staff at Human Kinetics (especially Loarn Robertson, Kevin Matz, Doug Fink, and their crews) and the models. Much gratitude to Karen Backstrom for her manuscript review and continued encouragement.

Finally, thanks to my patients. I have learned and continue to learn something from each of you every day. I hope I have, in return, given the knowledge of how to manage your injuries for life.

DVD CONTENTS

Introduction

Ankle and Foot Techniques

Arch Taping: Low Dye, Cross X, and Navicular Lift
Subtalar Neutral Stirrup Ankle Support
Calcaneus Inversion Glide
Calcaneus Inversion: Alternative Technique
Achilles Unloading
Hypermobile Distal Fibula
Hallux Abductovalgus (HAV) Bunion Correction
First Metatarsal–Cuneiform Glide
Fifth Metatarsal Dorsal Glide
Fifth Metatarsal–Cuboid Dorsal and Plantar Glide
Gastrocnemius Unloading

Knee Techniques

Patellar Medial Glide (Plus Tilt Corrections)
Patellar Tendon Unloading
Infrapatellar Fat Pad Unloading
Pes Anserinus Bursitis Unloading
Iliotibial Band Friction Syndrome
Proximal Fibular Glide
Tibiofemoral Torsion
Knee Hyperextension Block
Tensor Fascia Lata Glide
Medial Hamstring Unloading

Cervical, Thoracic, and Lumbopelvic Techniques

Postural Taping: Upper Back and Neck
Postural Taping: Midthoracic and Lumbar Areas
Postural Taping: Thoracic Vertebra Glide
Rib Support
Low Back Hyperextension Limit
Sacroiliac Joint Approximation
Ilial Shear, Anterior
Diamond Box Unloading
Hip and Gluteal Muscle Approximation

Shoulder Techniques

Elbow, Wrist, and Hand Techniques

Credits

Introduction to Taping

The proposed therapeutic effects of taping include stabilizing joints, changing and controlling posture at a joint, inhibiting muscle activity, reducing pain, increasing motor neuron excitability, and increasing joint torque. Taping has also been reported to enhance proprioception. Potential benefits include improved muscle effort, improved sensorimotor control, cutaneous stimulation, pain modulation, and facilitation or inhibition of muscle activity (Lewis, Wright, and Green 2005).

Texts on taping focus primarily on the use of athletic tape, and the taping techniques target athletic trainers and athletic training students. Some texts also explain Kinesio taping techniques. *Strap Taping for Sports and Rehabilitation* demonstrates use of (brown) strapping tape with a base of (white) tape, products more commonly used by physical therapists for treatment and prevention of injuries but available to the general public. Commonly used strapping tape techniques in physical therapy have been developed by Jenny McConnell, PT, and Brian Mulligan, PT, among others. Their philosophy is that tape is an adjunct to physical therapy treatment. The taping techniques presented in this book can be used to decrease pain, improve faulty biomechanics, diagnose which anatomical structures could be contributing to the symptoms, prevent further injury or pain, and more quickly return the patient to desired activity.

RELATIONSHIP BETWEEN TAPING AND ANATOMY

Tape has the benefit of acting directly on superficial structures through applied force or pressure, sometimes better than an off-the-shelf or custom brace. A good example is using tape to apply a medial force to the patella to change a laterally tracking patella into a more neutrally tracking one; this often decreases symptoms when a patellar cutout knee brace is not of benefit. Another example is creating pressure on a tight muscle or the Achilles tendon with tape to decrease symptoms of Achilles tendinitis or to physically change the location or alter joint (such as gliding of the distal fibula after an ankle sprain, thus decreasing lateral ankle pain).

TYPES OF TAPE

Let's compare the three types of tape: strapping tape, athletic tape, and Kinesio tape (see table 1.1).

Athletic tape (figure 1.1) can limit abnormal or excessive movement, provide support to muscles, enhance proprioceptive feedback, and secure protective pads (Perrin 2005), but it has a very short duration of effectiveness (20 minutes). It is applied immediately before an activity or sport and removed immediately afterward.

Leukotape and other similar brands of strapping tape (figure 1.2) have only a 30% stretch from the time of initial application and are therefore more useful for creating bracing support to the specific body area. This lack of stretch is especially important if the person is engaged in physical activity or a sport and is relying on the tape for stability. Strapping tape is very adherent (similar to duct tape) and can tear skin when applied directly, so a stretchy underwrap is usually applied first. The underwrap also serves as a force anchor instead of the bare skin. The tape can be left in place anywhere from 2 days to 1 week, through showering, until it loses its effect.

The other form of therapeutic taping uses Kinesio tape (figure 1.3), which has elasticity of up to 140% of the tape's original length. Kinesio tape allows full joint motion and works to aid lymphatic flow. It is applied directly to the skin without an underwrap. It is applied differently from athletic or strapping tape, often by taking a joint actively through its range of motion while applying the tape over the muscle or its antagonist, depending on whether the goal is to inhibit or facilitate muscle contraction. Kinesio tape, like strapping tape, can be worn for extended periods (up to 10 days) and withstands showering.

Despite its popularity, evidence for the effectiveness of Kinesio taping as the only treatment technique for an injury is limited, conflicting, and not of high quality (Thelen, Dauber, and Stoneman 2008; Vanti et al. 2007; Gonzalez-Iglesias et al. 2009; Garcia-Muro, Rodríguez-Fernández, and Herrero-de-Lucas 2009; Fu et al. 2008; Hsu et al. 2009). Kinesio taping was found to be effective in reducing pain, or increasing range of motion, or changing electromyographic activity only when used in conjunction with other physical therapy treatments such as manual therapy and exercise in persons with neurological problems such as stroke or cerebral palsy as well as in persons with orthopedic injuries (Adamczyk et al. 2009; Farrell, Naber, and Geigleet 2010; Hadala and Barrios 2009; Jaraczewska and Long 2006; Yasukawa, Patel, and Sisung 2006).

WHY STRAPPING TAPE?

Studies have shown that traditional athletic tape fails to support the area it is applied to after 20 minutes of physical activity (Bragg et al. 2002). In another study, using underwrap and rigid strapping tape gave better adhesion than traditional ankle athletic taping as well as enabled the

TABLE 1.1

Comparing Types of Tape

Type, uses	Examples of brand names	Underwrap	Elasticity	Applied by	Duration worn
Athletic tape Acute injury treatment, prevention of injury during sports activities, restricts some movement, relieves swelling	Johnson & Johnson, Cramer, Mueller	Underwrap or skin protectant required	Inelastic: failure after 20 minutes of use	ATCs, PTs, coaches, athletes, others with training	Varies: applied immediately before and removed immediately after activity or sport
Strapping tape Restricts some movement, helps correct postural or biomechanical faults, limits painful movement	Mueller Leukotape Endura-Tape DonJoy	Cover-Roll, Hypafix, Fixomull, or none	30% original length	PTs, PTAs, OTs, COTAs, some ATCs, others with training	48 hours to 7 days
Kinesio tape Allows for full joint movement in sport, assists with lymphatic drainage, relieves swelling and bruising, helps release myofascial restrictions	Balance-Tex Sports-Tex Kinesio-Tex Mueller	Not needed	140% original length	ATCs, PTs, chiropractors, certified Kinesio taping practitioners, others with training	3-10 days

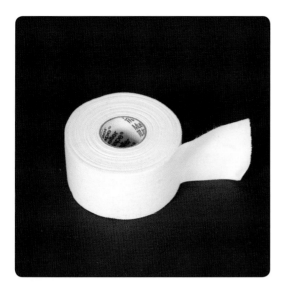

Figure 1.1 Athletic tape.

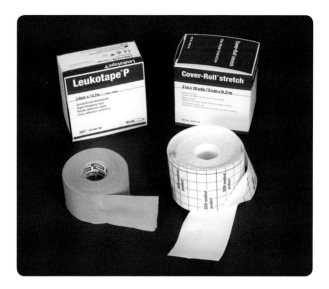

Figure 1.2 Leukotape (strapping tape); Cover-Roll (underwrap).

subject to withstand longer periods of athletic activity (Passerallo & Calabrese 1994).

The proper application of strapping tape provides the following benefits:

- An earlier return to desired activities and function (Whittingham, Palmer, and MacMillan 2004; Vicenzino et al. 2003; Alexander et al. 2003)

- The limitation of painful movement and the restoration of pain-free movement (Conway et al. 1992; Bockrath, Malone, and Conway 1993; Cushnagan, McCarthy, and Dieppe 1994; Cerny 1995; Powers et al. 1997; Gilleard, McConnell, and Parsons 1998; Cowan et al. 2002; Franettovich et al. 2008; Whittingham, Palmer, and MacMillan 2004; Ancliffe 1992; Morin and Bravo 1997; Warden et al. 2008; Vicenzino et al. 2003; Ng & Cheng 2002, 2009; Hinman et al. 2003; Herrington 2001, 2004, 2009; Hyland et al. 2006; Christou 2004; Richmond et al. 2009; Quilty et al. 2003; Crossley et al. 2001, 2002; Wilson, Carter, and Thomas 2003; McConnell 2000, 2002; Bennell et al. 2007; Host 1995; Lewis, Wright, and Green 2005; Shamus and Shamus 1997; Alexander et al. 2003; Moiler, Hall, and Robinson 2006; Peterson 2004)

- Mechanical support and joint stabilization (Peterson 2004; Meier et al. 2008; Lange,

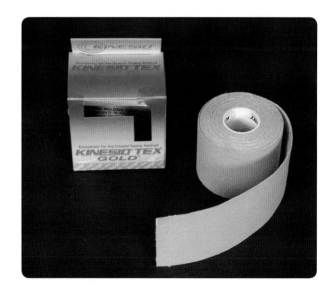

Figure 1.3 Kinesio tape.

Chipchase, and Evans 2004; Delahunt, O'Driscoll, and Moran 2009; Crossley et al. 2009; Nolan et al. 2009; Herrington and Al-Shebli 2006; Alexander et al. 2003; Lewis, Wright, and Green 2005; McConnell 2002)

- Correction of postural or joint alignment (Lewis, Wright, and Green 2005; Host 1995; Crossley et al. 2009; Herrington 2004, 2009; Hyland et al. 2006; Peterson 2004; Morin and Bravo 1997; Van de Water and Speksnijder 2010; Schoffel et al 2007;

Bennell et al. 2007; Adams and Madden 2009; Hyland et al. 2006; Carter and Chockalingam 2009; Lange, Chipchase, and Evans 2004; Nolan et al. 2009; Franettovich et al. 2008)

- Facilitation or inhibition of muscles (Alexander et al. 2003; Tobin and Robinson 2000; Gilleard, McConnell, and Parsons 1998; Carda and Molteni 2005; Ernst, Kawaguchi, and Saliba 1999; Herrington 2001; Maguire et al. 2010; Lewis, Wright, and Green 2005; Iosa et al. 2009; Hall et al. 1995; Kilbreath et al. 2006; Miller and Osmotherly 2009)
- Improved proprioception (Hughes and Rochester 2008; Alexander et al. 2003)
- An extension of manual therapy techniques or improved accessory joint mobility (Alexander et al. 2003; Vicenzino 2003; Vicenzino, Paungmali, and Teys 2007; Shamus and Shamus 1997; Adams and Madden 2009; Mulligan 1999)
- The management and treatment of joint hypermobility syndrome (Simmonds and Keer 2007)

TAPING GUIDELINES

The first step is to accurately assess what causes or contributes to the symptoms; this is especially important in light of the activity the patient wishes to perform. For example, if someone is having anterior knee pain and has a sedentary lifestyle, the approach to treatment may be taping the knee first to allow for pain-free basic strengthening of the leg. To treat anterior knee pain in a marathoner who has flat feet, however, my approach may be to tape the feet and ankles first to see the effect proper leg posture has on decreasing the anterior knee pain.

Taping is used as an adjunct to other treatment options, including

- exercise for muscle imbalances;
- the stretching of tight muscles;
- postural retraining;
- biomechanical evaluation and education of proper form during the aggravating activity;

- manual physical therapy to address joint and soft-tissue restrictions; and
- modalities such as ice, heat, and electrical stimulation (for pain control or muscle reeducation) used in physical therapy.

Once you define your goal for applying the tape, a good knowledge of anatomy and biomechanics is imperative in choosing the proper technique to use.

Scope of Practice

Athletic trainers are trained in athletic taping, and physical therapists may or may not have been trained in strap taping. Note that there is a difference. Many athletic taping techniques can be modified (i.e., to use less tape) to a strapping tape application. Strapping tape is more rigid and can provide more long-lasting support, with the specific goal of bracing the area, enhancing manual therapy techniques, and enhancing or inhibiting muscle contraction. Patients and their family members can be instructed in how to tape effectively by watching the physical therapist demonstrate the technique and the purpose of the tape. Taping is a creative process as long as the precautions are kept in mind and the patient's pain or symptoms decrease when the tape is applied. Do not rely on taping alone to assist in the assessment and treatment of injuries; a thorough evaluation by a qualified health professional is an essential first step in determining appropriate treatment options.

Taping Precautions

There are several precautions to be aware of when taping. Some are covered here.

Allergy to Latex or Adhesives

Most underwrap products do not contain latex, whereas Leukotape and other brands of strapping tape do. These can usually be applied to persons with a latex allergy without problems as long as the strapping tape does not directly contact the skin. If a person has a skin allergy or sensitivity to either latex or adhesives, a red raised rash will appear directly under the tape and may be very itchy. Blisters may also be present. An allergy will usually occur within the first 24 hours after application.

It is common for the skin to be red immediately after the tape is removed, especially if the tape has been on the skin for a long time. This usually fades within a few minutes to a few hours. Cortisone or other topical anti-inflammatory creams can soothe skin irritation. Spreading a liquid antacid or milk of magnesia over the affected skin area or using a skin protectant before applying tape can also be helpful. If the skin is sensitive or irritated, tape for only short periods.

Friction Rub or Blistering

Friction can occur when the tape exerts a forceful pull on the skin or under a piece of anchor tape (which is a piece of either underwrap or strapping tape that is applied to secure other pieces of tape). Tension or excessive movement (most commonly seen around the anterior knee) can cause skin to break down and tear. If the client complains of pain in a localized area under the tape, remove the tape carefully and slowly. Skin in this area will toughen with time and be less susceptible to breakdown.

Limited Range of Motion at a Joint

Be aware of the range of motion required for the activity the patient wants to perform. The tape should be applied so that it does not limit joint mobility or inhibit performance.

Impaired Circulation Distal to the Taped Area

When taping completely around a joint (elbow, knee, ankle, wrist), ensure that the tape isn't so tight that it impairs circulation to the area distal to the tape. Tightness can impede venous return and create swelling in the hand or foot as well as cause more serious complications.

Fragile Skin

Take caution when taping persons with delicate skin (e.g., elderly, children, patients with connective tissue disorders, people with diabetes prone to skin breakdown) or when taping over open or scabbed wounds or over recent or not fully closed surgical scars. It is possible to tape over a bandage covering an open wound or scab and

---

The following supplies are needed for taping:

Rubbing alcohol
Underwrap of choice
Strapping tape of choice
Razor if area is hairy
Scissors
Adhesive remover

---

have patients wear the tape for shorter periods so the wound status can be checked. A small test strip of underwrap tape worn on the skin for 2 or 3 days to see how it is tolerated is advised in those with skin integrity issues.

Excessive Hair

Tape sticks better directly to bare skin. The more hair in the area, the more difficult it is to keep the tape on (not to mention the agony of pulling the tape off along with the hair underneath it!). Ensure the patient has shaved the area to be taped; otherwise taping will not be as successful.

TAPING APPLICATION

Here are the general steps to consider when taping. Store tape at room temperature. Excessive heat will make the strapping tape difficult to pull from the roll.

1. Decide the purpose of taping (e.g., to increase or decrease range of motion, to decrease pain, to improve function) and where the tape should be placed. Perform any screening tests to assess for taping efficacy with decrease in symptoms.

2. Prepare the area to be taped: Make sure the skin is shaved, clean (wipe with rubbing alcohol if skin appears dirty or oily), and free of residual adhesive from prior taping (use adhesive remover); remove clothing that impairs access to the area to be taped.

3. Position the patient in a way that allows you best access to the body part and the best neutral anatomical position for applying the tape. Normally for any taping technique superior to the thoracolumbar junction, tape with the patient in a sitting position; for taping the lumbar spine and distal, the patient should be prone, supine, or standing. The back or pelvis is usually taped with the subject standing. Some techniques require two clinicians to be most effective.

4. Measure and cut strips of underwrap, and apply enough that the strapping tape will not contact the skin (except in the case of taping the foot, where underwrap is optional).

5. Cut strips of strapping tape, and apply with adequate tension in the desired direction of pull to create some wrinkling in the underwrap and sometimes wrinkling or gathering of the skin (figure 1.4).

6. Assess the integrity of the tape by taking the joint through a range of motion necessary for the activity the patient will perform (e.g., for a taped knee, have the patient bend and straighten her knee; for a taped foot, have them walk). You may need to apply pressure to the ends of the tape if the edges start to pull loose, or add anchor strips of underwrap to the ends of the taping strips to secure them (especially around the knee) (figure 1.5).

7. Assess for pain control or changes in symptoms. The tape should quickly do its job and decrease pain when the patient moves in a way that previously caused pain (e.g., taping the foot should immediately improve heel or arch pain upon walking). Sometimes it may be necessary to reapply the tape or change the angle or force of pull. If the strapping tape does not improve symptoms or causes pain in another area, it should be removed.

8. Depending on skin tolerance and the tape's integrity, strapping tape can remain intact for 2 to 7 days through showers and sweating. Swimming or excessive exposure to water will decrease adherence time. Oily or very sweaty skin will also decrease adherence time, especially on the foot. Tape edges will become ragged and can start to peel off. When there is no longer enough tension or symptoms start to return, it is time to remove the tape.

The patient must continue to wear tape until the muscles are strong enough to support the area during activity and have the endurance to maintain the position for the desired time. Typically if symptoms are acute, the tape is worn for 3 to 5 days during normal activity; once pain is diminished, the patient slowly incorporates the aggravating or sporting activity into his day, wearing tape only during this particular activity. It could take from days to weeks to months to return to regular activities, depending on

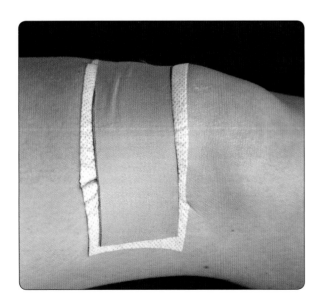

Figure 1.4 Tension of the strapping tape causing underwrap wrinkling.

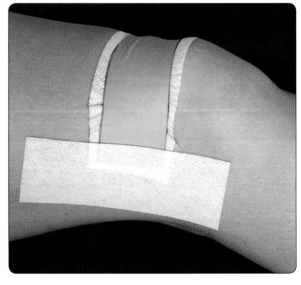

Figure 1.5 Anchor strips using underwrap.

compliance with strengthening exercises and the patient's attention to correction of faulty biomechanics during the activity. Most of the time, when muscle strength and endurance have improved, the tape will no longer need to be used. However, good biomechanics must be used forever. If a patient's poor form may be contributing to her symptoms, they may need to be instructed in proper form.

9. To remove the tape, start peeling it off at an edge of the underwrap; peel slowly so as not to tear the skin. Removal is easiest when the tape and skin are wet, such as after a shower, bath, or swim. For foot taping where no underwrap is used, pull a strip away from the skin, and carefully cut through that strip so it can be removed.

DOCUMENTATION

For clinical documentation or charting purposes, list the taping technique used and the aim of the technique. It may be helpful to note if extra strapping pieces were added for support. Generally, the time billed for taping includes the time it takes to prep the area to be taped, apply the tape, and assess efficacy of the taping technique when the patient performs certain symptom-aggravating movements. This time frame can range from 5 to 15 minutes depending on the size of the area, the efficiency of the therapist, and whether a second therapist is needed to assist in applying the tape. In the United States, the 15-minute charge codes commonly used in physical therapy are manual therapy, neuromuscular reeducation, and strapping (when covered by insurance).

Ankle and Foot

The ankle and foot have minimal muscle bulk or adipose tissue (except on the plantar surface of the foot); thus this area can be influenced quite dramatically when superficial joints (such as the tibiofibular and midfoot joints) are taped. Taping helps correct ankle and distal fibula position, encourages correct muscle activation, and provides support to the joints and arch without the bulk of an ankle brace. The restriction offered by strapping tape may prevent movement to the end of the joint's range of motion, where injury may be most likely to occur; adhesive strapping for the ankle must provide support to the talocrural and subtalar joints to be most effective (Ator et al. 1991). Taping the foot is sometimes essential for clients involved in activities in which they are barefoot (such as gymnastics, yoga, or Pilates) or if they use shoes with limited support (such as ballet slippers or jazz shoes for a dancer) or shoes that cannot accommodate a brace (e.g., tight-fitting shoes such as cleats, wrestling shoes, or dress shoes).

As we age, our arches tend to fall because the cumulative effects of gravity and weight bearing cause increased pronation of the foot and changes in biomechanical forces that can lead to problems such as pain and tendinitis. Choosing the proper supportive shoe specific to the activity is essential. The techniques I most commonly use with both active patients who engage in activities without shoes and the general patient population with ankle and foot problems are arch taping plus the stirrup technique. Clients should notice an immediate and beneficial difference as soon as they stand on the taped ankle or foot.

The following techniques are covered in this chapter: three types of arch taping (low Dye, cross X, navicular lift), stirrup, Achilles unloading, hypermobile distal fibula, hallux abductovalgus (HAV) (bunion) correction, first metatarsal–cuneiform glide, fifth metatarsal dorsal glide, cuboid glide, calcaneal glide, and gastrocnemius unloading. Orthotics appropriateness and footwear recommendations are also discussed.

Treatments are described for the following problems: heel spurs and pain; plantar fasciitis; Morton's neuroma; shin splints; midfoot sprain or pain; medial tibial stress syndrome; metatarsalgia; tarsal tunnel syndrome; foot alignment issues contributing to medial knee, hip, and low back pain (LBP); ankle or foot tendinitis; "fallen arches" (pronated feet); tarsal coalition; calcaneal bursitis; ankle fracture rehabilitation; Achilles tendinitis or partial tears; Sever's disease; chronic lateral or medial ankle pain or sprains; bunions; plantar ligament injury (toe hyperflexion); and turf toe (lateral collateral ligament or hyperextension injury).

If the ankle or foot is hairy, make sure the client shaves before tape application to ensure good adhesion. And make sure the area to be taped is clean. Start with brown strapping tape; if the skin is frail or sensitive, apply underwrap first. Tape may not adhere well if the client sweats a lot, so strapping tape only is preferred for the foot techniques so the tape will adhere longer.

ANATOMY OF THE ANKLE AND FOOT

The ankle mortise is made up of the distal tibia, fibula, talus (talocrural joint), subtalar joint (talus and calcaneus), talocalcaneonavicular joint, and calcaneocuboid joint. Ankle position can be affected by the ligamentous stability, musculotendinous lengths, and position of the bones and joints of the foot, such as the navicular height, medial arch height, tarsometatarsal joint, midtarsal joint, metatarsophalangeal (MTP) joint, and interphalangeal (IP) joint. The ankle and foot play a critical role in proprioception to maintain balance, especially during activities performed on uneven surfaces. During dynamic activities where the heel is off the ground (running, jumping, walking), the ankle can be vulnerable to strains and sprains because the base of support is smaller (just the ball of the foot instead of the entire plantar surface).

EVIDENCE

Taping and decreased pronation of the foot. Clinicians use strapping tape to temporarily control pronation of the foot and treat pain and conditions related to excessive pronation. Ralph Dye first described high-Dye and low-Dye taping, which are two common forms of strap taping. Low-Dye taping is applied to the foot only; it supports the medial longitudinal arch and reduces excessive foot pronation. High-Dye taping extends from the foot up to the distal leg (tibia and fibula) to provide support to an unstable ankle, prevent excessive ankle mobility, and counter the medial forces associated with excessive pronation (Carter and Chockalingam 2009).

In a review of the literature, Franettovich et al. (2008) found that antipronation tape has the biomechanical effect of increasing navicular height and medial longitudinal arch height, reducing tibial internal rotation and calcaneal eversion, and altering plantar pressure patterns under both static and dynamic conditions. The reduction in pronation ranged from a 5% increase in longitudinal arch height during jogging to as much as a 33% change in calcaneal eversion during walking.

Previous literature suggests that the increase in arch height with taping is likely clinically

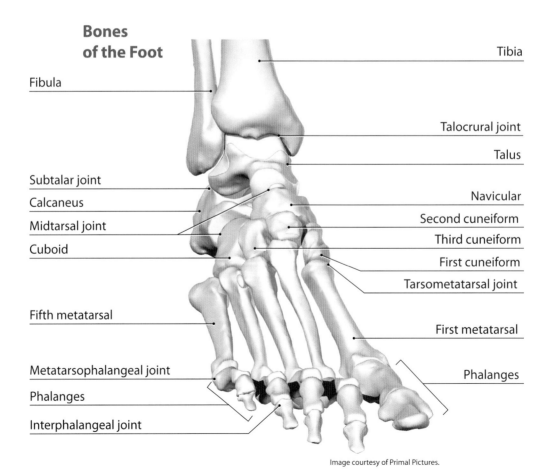

Bones of the Foot

Fibula

Subtalar joint

Calcaneus

Midtarsal joint

Cuboid

Fifth metatarsal

Metatarsophalangeal joint

Phalanges

Interphalangeal joint

Tibia

Talocrural joint

Talus

Navicular

Second cuneiform

Third cuneiform

First cuneiform

Tarsometatarsal joint

First metatarsal

Phalanges

Image courtesy of Primal Pictures.

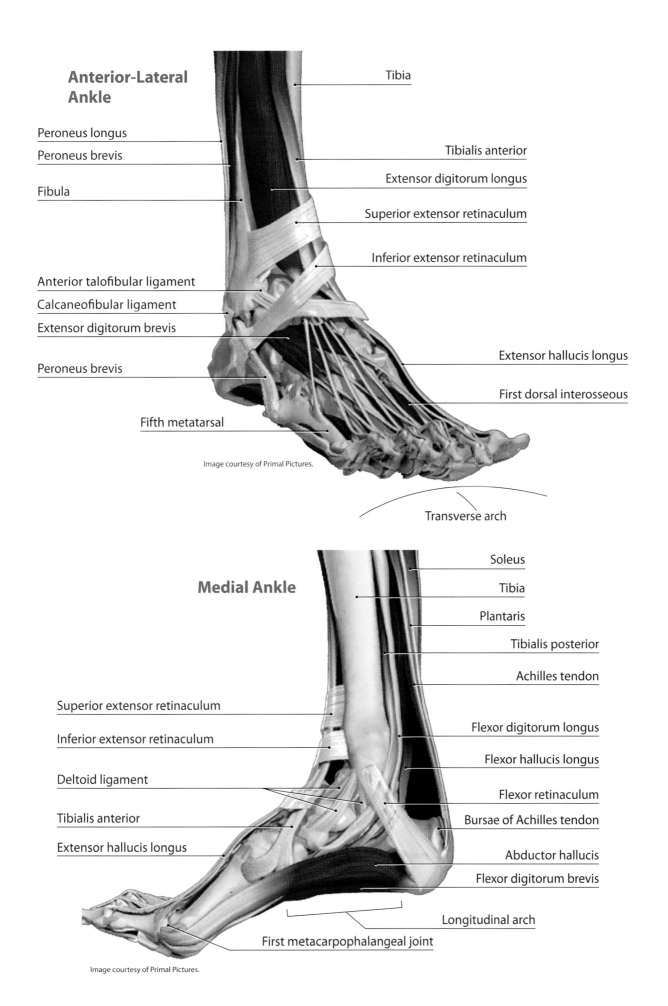

Anterior-Lateral Ankle

Peroneus longus

Peroneus brevis

Fibula

Anterior talofibular ligament

Calcaneofibular ligament

Extensor digitorum brevis

Peroneus brevis

Fifth metatarsal

Tibia

Tibialis anterior

Extensor digitorum longus

Superior extensor retinaculum

Inferior extensor retinaculum

Extensor hallucis longus

First dorsal interosseous

Image courtesy of Primal Pictures.

Transverse arch

Medial Ankle

Superior extensor retinaculum

Inferior extensor retinaculum

Deltoid ligament

Tibialis anterior

Extensor hallucis longus

Soleus

Tibia

Plantaris

Tibialis posterior

Achilles tendon

Flexor digitorum longus

Flexor hallucis longus

Flexor retinaculum

Bursae of Achilles tendon

Abductor hallucis

Flexor digitorum brevis

Longitudinal arch

First metacarpophalangeal joint

Image courtesy of Primal Pictures.

Posterior Muscles

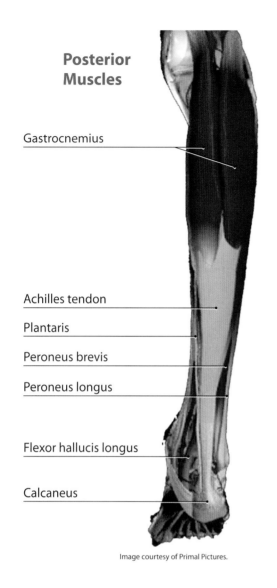

Gastrocnemius

Achilles tendon

Plantaris

Peroneus brevis

Peroneus longus

Flexor hallucis longus

Calcaneus

Image courtesy of Primal Pictures.

Surface Anatomy

Tibia

Tibialis anterior

Flexor digitorum longus

Medial malleolus

Sustentaculum tali

Abductor hallucis

Tuberosity of navicular

Head of first metatarsal

Extensor hallucis longus

Extensor digitorum longus

Image courtesy of Primal Pictures.

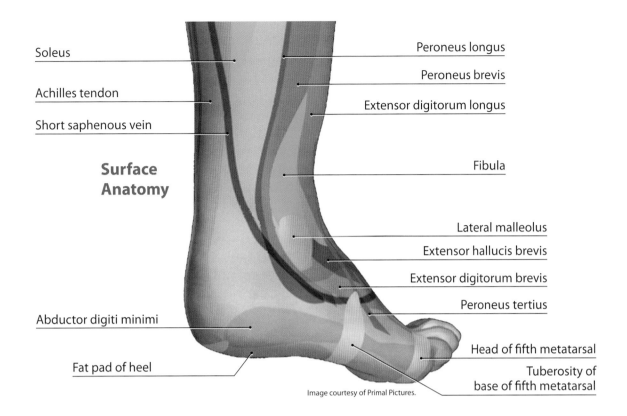

Surface Anatomy

Soleus

Achilles tendon

Short saphenous vein

Peroneus longus

Peroneus brevis

Extensor digitorum longus

Fibula

Lateral malleolus

Extensor hallucis brevis

Extensor digitorum brevis

Peroneus tertius

Abductor digiti minimi

Fat pad of heel

Head of fifth metatarsal

Tuberosity of base of fifth metatarsal

Image courtesy of Primal Pictures.

relevant and may contribute to the benefit of arch tape in the treatment of lower extremity pain and injury. Continual use of an augmented low-Dye taping technique for approximately 12 days produced a small change in foot posture (Franettovich et al. 2009).

In a study by Lange, Chipchase, and Evans (2004), low-Dye taping significantly altered plantar pressure values in subjects with navicular drop of more than 10 mm. Peak and mean plantar pressure increased under the lateral midfoot and under the toes and decreased under the heel and forefoot, suggesting a decrease in the amount of pronation. An augmented low-Dye technique also produced significant increases in lateral midfoot plantar pressures (Vicenzino, McPoil, and Buckland 2007), and similar results were shown by Russo and Chipchase (2001). In another study by Nolan et al. (2009), asymptomatic subjects with excessive pronation (defined as navicular drop greater than 10 mm) were taped with the low-Dye technique. The initial effect of reduced lateral forefoot peak plantar pressure was lost after a 10-minute walk, but the tape continued to have an effect on the medial forefoot after 20 minutes of exercise.

Taping and muscle facilitation. Taping also provides support to weak muscles, facilitating their normal activity. In a study by Iosa et al. (2009), improvements in gait pattern occurred during the taping treatment period and were then maintained, without further changes, in the 6 months after the study. Preliminary evidence suggests that antipronation tape reduces the activity of several muscles of the leg during dynamic activities (45% for tibialis posterior) (Franettovich et al. 2008).

Taping and joint position correction. A cuboid subluxation can occur from a forceful inversion injury to the foot, with patient complaints of midlateral foot pain. Adams and Madden (2009) recommend taping the foot after cuboid subluxation along with other conservative measures, such as cuboid manipulation, bracing, activity modification, and orthotics. Most athletes and dancers return to full participation after successful treatment.

In a study by Hopper et al. (2009), Mulligan lateral ankle taping did not influence performance during static and dynamic balance activities in subjects with unilateral chronic ankle instability under resting and fatigued conditions.

Delahunt et al. (2010) found that fibular repositioning taping or lateral subtalar sling taping did not affect dynamic ankle stability, but the participants' perceived confidence and stability did improve.

Taping is also effective in correcting dysfunction with superficial joint-gliding manual techniques, such as mobilization with movement. "Mobilization with movement (MWM) is a manual therapy treatment technique in which a manual force, usually in the form of a joint glide, is applied to a motion segment and sustained while a previously impaired action (e.g., painful reduced movement, painful muscle contraction) is performed. The technique is indicated if, during its application the technique enables the impaired joint to move freely without pain or impediment. The direction of the applied force (translation or rotation) is typically perpendicular to the plane of movement or impaired action and in some instances it is parallel to the treatment plane" (Mulligan 1999). These techniques are used quite commonly, and taping is an effective way to maintain joint position correction once it is attained with mobilization.

Taping and proprioception. The literature on taping is limited in terms of quantity and methodological quality in relation to taping's effect on muscle reaction time, kinesthesia, and postural sway (Hughes and Rochester 2008).

Taping and joint stability. In a study by Alt, Lohrer, and Gollhofer (1999), approxi-

---

Footwear

A change in footwear can improve foot, ankle, and some knee, hip, and back symptoms or pain complaints. Footwear modification plus orthotics can make a significant improvement in many of the remaining cases. Patients' shoes should be inspected if they have been worn for a length of time; the pattern of wear on the sole and deformation of the upper material of the shoe may indicate whether joint biomechanics are normal or abnormal. See McPoil's 1988 article, "Footwear" in *Physical Therapy* for more information.

Footwear design has an effect on ground reaction forces and foot and leg kinematics. Specific shoe characteristics may be indicated based on the patient's problems. For a foot that is hypermobile or excessively pronated (fallen arch) during standing and weight-bearing activities, a stiff-soled shoe may help control foot hypermobility and thus decrease symptoms.

Shoes that are soft, flexible, and easily torsioned (figure 2.1*a-b*) may be desirable for managing problems associated with hypomobile or excessively supinated (high arch, rigid) feet. Any deformation of the shoe during weight bearing will assist in dispersing the ground reaction forces and may compensate for the inability of the hypomobile foot to do so. Soles that are too soft may deform too quickly during loading, resulting in a greater ground reaction force and possibly an increase in symptoms (McPoil, 1988).

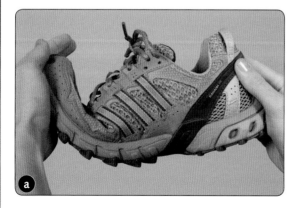 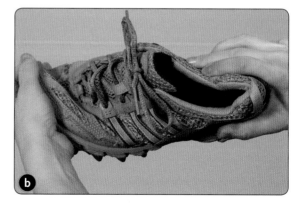

Figure 2.1 Shoe stiffness (*a*) and torsion (*b*) tests.

mately 35% of initial maximum inversion was decreased by ankle taping. Depending on the technique, there was a loss of tape stability greater or equal to 14% after 30 minutes of exercise. The improved joint stability was due to mechanical stiffness of the tape application. Joint stability was influenced positively by neuromuscular proprioceptive and physiological processes, as demonstrated by increased electromyographic activation.

The results of a study by Delahunt, O'Driscoll, and Moran (2009) indicate that ankle taping reduced the degree of plantar flexion immediately before and at initial contact with the ground, and these reductions were retained even after exercise. A study by Herrington and Al-Shebli (2006) indicates that prophylactic strap taping, though restricting range of movement, does not affect vertical jump performance.

Taping and decreased pain and increased function. Calcaneal taping is a more effective tool for the relief of plantar heel pain than stretching, sham taping (taping that for the purpose of the study does not alter joint mechanics), or no treatment (Hyland et al. 2006). Alexander et al. (2003) showed that taping in addition to stretching exercises has added value, and there is limited evidence that taping can reduce pain short term in patients with plantar fasciosis. In a study by Osborne and Allison (2006), treatment of plantar fasciitis by low-Dye taping and iontophoresis with acetic acid for 4 weeks was the preferred option.

ORTHOTICS

In a study by Meier et al. (2008), athletes with lower extremity foot pain caused by overuse were taped for 3 days. If the taping was effective, foot orthotics (figure 2.2a-b) were fabricated. After wearing the foot orthotics for 4 weeks, all athletes reported a substantial reduction in their pain and an increase in function. These results indicate that changes in foot posture created by taping can be used to guide foot orthosis prescription. I use the arch taping with stirrup technique combination to determine if orthotics would be beneficial for patients. If pain is decreased, orthotics are recommended.

According to Vicenzino (2004, abstract), "the clinical efficacy, mechanical effects, and underlying mechanism of the action of foot orthotics has not been conclusively determined making it difficult for practitioners to agree on a reliable and valid clinical approach to their application and even their fabrication. This problem is compounded by evidence suggesting that the most commonly used approach for orthotic prescription (*Biomechanical Evaluation of the Foot*. Vol. 1. Clinical Biomechanics Corporation, Los Angeles, 1971) has poor validity and many of the associated clinical measurements of that approach lack adequate levels of reliability." He outlines a new approach that is "based on two key elements. One is the identification, verification and quantification of physical tasks that serve as client specific outcome measures. The second is the application of specific physical manipulations during the performance of these physical tasks. The physical manipulations are selected on the basis of motion dysfunction, and their immediate effects on the client specific outcome measures serve as the basis to making an informed decision on the propriety of using orthotics in individual clients. The motion dysfunction also guides the type of orthotic that is applied" (2004, abstract). I have dealt with many frustrated clients who had spent a lot of money on custom orthotics that did not improve their pain. Thanks to a thorough evaluation, these clients now have improved symptoms due to a change in choice of shoe, a change in custom orthotic, or use of an off-the-shelf orthotic.

More than 50% of the literature suggests orthotics are used for motion control, but this is backed by little evidence. There are two theories for using foot orthotics: balanced foot and total contact (McPoil and Cornwall 2007). The balanced foot theory is based on maintaining subtalar joint neutral during activities. Foot alignment is evaluated while the subject is not bearing weight, and deformities (e.g., forefoot varus or valgus, rearfoot varus) are corrected using forefoot or rearfoot wedges or posts. The problem with this theory is that the subtalar joint does not function about the neutral position during walking, and assessment tests for

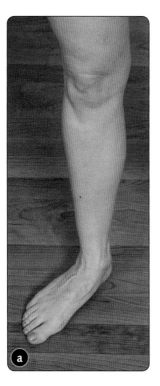 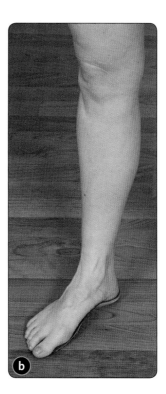

Figure 2.2 Lower extremity positioning (*a*) before and (*b*) after custom orthotics.

biomechanics have poor interrater reliability both in palpating subtalar neutral and for testing procedures.

The total contact theory states that orthotics stabilize the medial and lateral longitudinal arches, permitting dynamic movement of the medial longitudinal arch but controlling motion to limit end-range movement. Density of the orthotic materials used for fabrication must permit dynamic but controlled midfoot and rearfoot motion. Evidence validates that the area of greatest pronation and supination is in the midfoot, and total contact provides improved arch stability. If motion control is the goal, then the orthotic should support the rearfoot and midfoot.

In motion studies, however, both balanced and total contact orthotics produce an average of greater than or equal to 2° control, and the density and firmness of materials appear to make no difference in regard to motion control (McPoil and Cornwall 2000; Genova and Gross 2000; Brown et al 1995; Gross 1995). So either method can be used when choosing orthotics, and cost may be the determining factor.

Orthotics can be helpful in treating cases of foot, ankle, knee, and sometimes hip and back pain. Depending on how much patients are willing to pay for custom orthotics (which require a mold or cast of the foot made by a physical therapist, orthotist, podiatrist, or other health professional), prices range from US$100 to $700 and sometimes even higher. If clients do not want to spend that kind of money, I may start them on an off-the-shelf product that can be obtained for as little as US$10. Superfeet provide a good selection of off-the-shelf orthotics (starting at US$35) tailored to the active population, with insert stiffness based on activity level. Standing force-plate imaging is becoming increasingly accessible (often found in the medical supply section of your local drugstore), but I have not found the orthotics generated or recommended by force-plate data alone to be as effective as casted orthotics.

EVALUATION

A thorough evaluation is required, including a proximal screen of the low back, hips, knees, and feet. Obtain results of any X-rays or imaging. Table 2.1 provides the normal active range of motion (AROM) of the ankle and foot (figure 2.3).

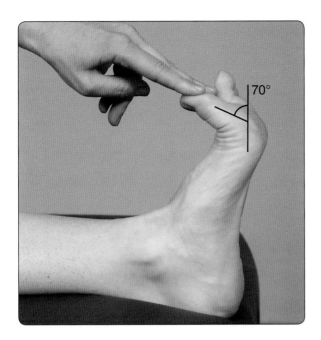

70°

Figure 2.3 First metatarsophalangeal joint range of motion.

Special Tests

Hypermobility of the ankle can be assessed with the anterior drawer test. The patient is supine, the ankle positioned in 10 to 15° of plantar flexion and the heel is pulled anteriorly while the tibia and fibula are stabilized; the test is positive if there is excessive anterior translation compared with the other ankle (Cleland 2007). Taping techniques that include the ankle (stirrup, high Dye) will be beneficial if the ankle is hypermobile.

Biomechanical Considerations

While the patient is walking, running, or performing another specific activity, observe the foot and ankle position, amount of pronation,

TABLE 2.1

Normal AROM of Ankle and Foot

Motion	Degree
Ankle dorsiflexion	20°
Ankle plantar flexion	50°
Ankle/foot supination	45-60°
Ankle/foot pronation	15-30°
1st MTP (big toe) extension	70°
2nd-4th MTP extension	40°

Adapted from Magee 2006

calcaneal varus or valgus, and forefoot varus or valgus as compared with neutral position.

● Have the patient perform a single-leg squat (see chapter 3 for details; page 56) (figure 2.4).

● Assess leg length (figure 2.5): With the patient prone, compare leg length at the malleoli; compare height of the tibias (figure 2.6) with the knees flexed 90°. Leg length discrepancy is present if the malleoli are unequal in prone; unequal tibia heights when the knees are flexed indicate a discrepancy in tibia length (Hertling and Kessler 1996). This can be validated in standing by assessing iliac crest heights for general leg length discrepancy (figure 2.7). Iliac length discrepancy can be assessed through palpation while lying prone (comparing distance between the iliac crest and ischial tuberosity, shown in figure 2.8) or sitting (comparing iliac crest height). Femur length can be assessed by palpating the distance between the greater trochanter and fibular head and comparing the measurements (figure 2.9).

● Determine the type of shoe the client is wearing, what surface the aggravating activity is performed on, and whether orthotics are used.

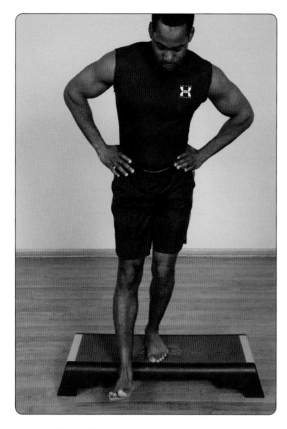

Figure 2.4 Single-leg squat observation: maintaining anatomical neutral.

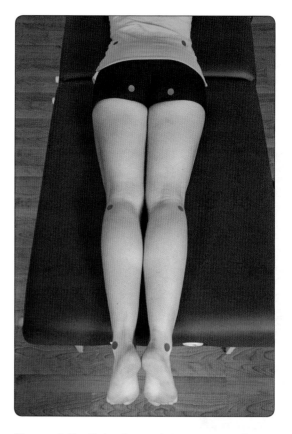

Figure 2.5 Palpation points to assess leg length discrepancy.

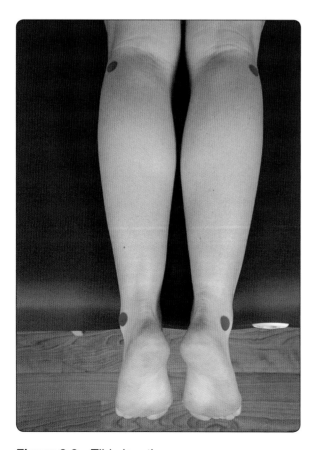

Figure 2.6 Tibia length.

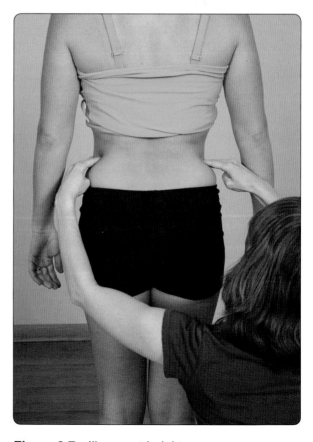

Figure 2.7 Iliac crest height.

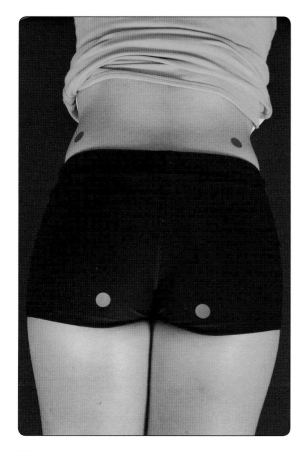

Figure 2.8 Ilia length.

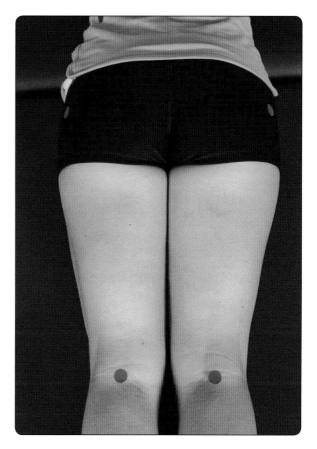

Figure 2.9 Femur length.

Technique	Screening tool
Achilles tendon unloading	Achilles tendon compression
Hypermobile distal fibula	Distal fibula accessory movement
First metatarsal—cuneiform glide	First metatarsal—cuneiform accessory movement
Fifth metatarsal—cuboid glide	Fifth metatarsal—cuboid accessory glides
Fifth metatarsal dorsal glide	Fifth metatarsal accessory movement
Cuboid glide	Cuboid accessory movement
Calcaneal inversion glide	Calcaneal accessory movement
Gastrocnemius unloading	Gastrocnemius medial/lateral glide
Orthotic recommendation	Arch taping (plus stirrup technique)

LOW DYE

Indications

This technique is effective for treating heel pain or spurs, plantar fasciitis, Morton's neuroma, shin splints, midfoot sprain or strain, medial tibial stress syndrome, metatarsalgia, tarsal tunnel syndrome, medial knee pain, and hip or low back pain. It is also used for clients who perform activities barefoot or in shoes that are tight or offer little support.

Client's Position

The client is prone with the foot hanging off the table; an alternate position is supine with the heel hanging off the table, ankle in 0° dorsiflexion and in subtalar neutral.

Physical Therapist's Position

The PT is sitting on a stool or chair at the end of the table.

Application Guidelines

1. While maintaining the rearfoot and forefoot position in the frontal plane, add the forefoot and plantar flexion of the first ray (the big toe and first metatarsal) while laying the spur strip of tape down on the medial side of the foot and around the heel to the lateral side of the foot, finishing proximal to the metatarsophalangeal joint (*a*).

2. Apply two to four strips of tape (mini-stirrups) to the medial longitudinal arch, starting from the lateral side of the foot and passing under the arch to the medial foot (*b*). An inversion force can be applied to the foot. The initial strip is just proximal to the metatarsal heads, progressing posteriorly and overlapping the other pieces of tape, with the last strip ending just distal to the tendon of the anterior tibialis; the plantar heel remains untaped.

3. End with an anchor strip over the dorsal aspect of the foot, just proximal to the metatarsal heads, making sure the tape does not impede toe motion (*c-d*).

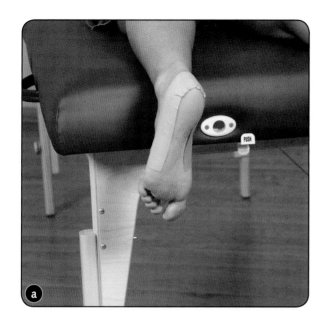

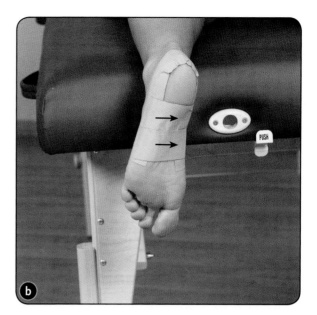

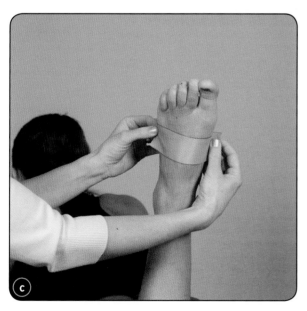

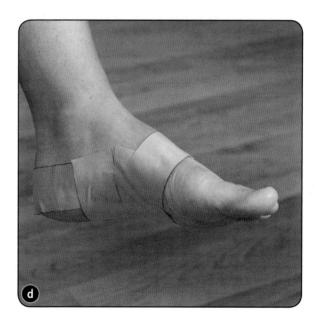

CROSS X

Indications

This technique is effective for treating heel pain or spurs, plantar fasciitis, Morton's neuroma, shin splints, midfoot sprain or strain, medial tibial stress syndrome, metatarsalgia, tarsal tunnel syndrome, medial knee pain, and hip or low back pain. It is also used for clients who perform activities barefoot or in shoes that are tight or offer little support.

Client's Position

The client is prone with the foot hanging off the table; an alternate position is supine with the heel hanging off the table, ankle in 0° dorsiflexion and in subtalar neutral.

Physical Therapist's Position

The PT is sitting on a stool or chair at the end of the table.

Application Guidelines (McPoil and McGarvey)

1. Cut a strip of adhesive tape in half (narrow width) and apply it, starting plantarly from the first metatarsal head and moving laterally around the posterior surface of the calcaneus and across the arch, attaching the tape to the plantar surface of the fifth metatarsal head (a).

2. Apply four more strips (two in each direction), overlapping the tape pieces by 1/4 inch (6 mm) (b).

3. Apply two to four strips of tape (mini-stirrups) to the medial longitudinal arch, starting from the lateral side of the foot and passing under the arch to the lateral foot. An inversion force can be applied to the foot. The initial strip goes just proximal to the metatarsal heads, progressing posteriorly and overlapping the other pieces of tape, with the last strip ending just distal to the tendon of the anterior tibialis; the plantar heel remains untaped (c).

4. While maintaining the rearfoot and forefoot position in the frontal plane, add the forefoot and plantar flexion of the first ray while laying the spur strip of tape down on the medial side of the foot and around the heel to the lateral side of the foot, finishing proximal to the metatarsophalangeal joint (d).

5. End with an anchor strip over the dorsal aspect of the foot, just proximal to the metatarsal heads, making sure the tape does not impede toe motion (see figure c of low dye technique on page 21).

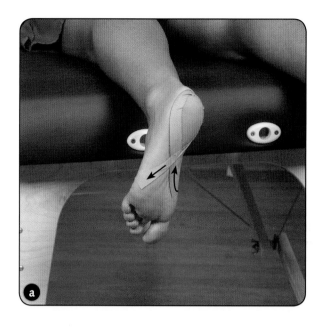

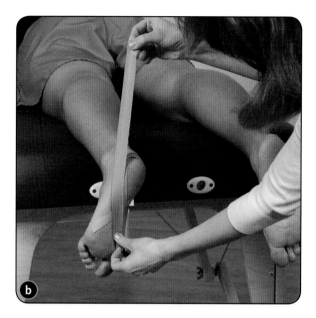

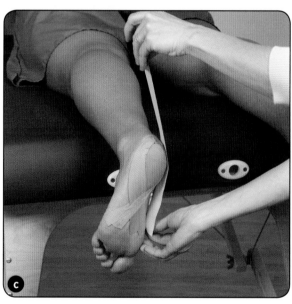

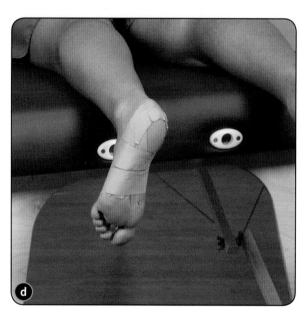

NAVICULAR LIFT

Indications

This technique is used to increase supination and stability of the foot.

Client's Position

The client is prone with the foot hanging off the table; an alternate position is supine with the heel hanging off the table, ankle in 0° dorsiflexion and in subtalar neutral.

Physical Therapist's Position

The PT is sitting on a stool or chair at the end of the table.

Application Guidelines (McConnell)

1. Start at the top of the foot in the area of the tarsometatarsal joints (*a*).
2. Apply strapping tape around the lateral foot. Pull with some force to supinate the foot and enhance the arch, and end medial to the Achilles tendon (*b*).

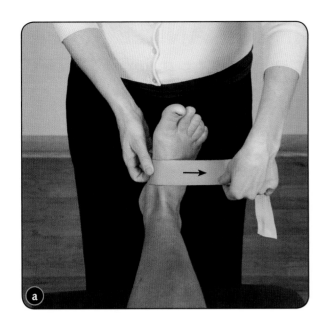 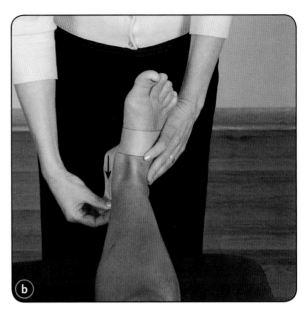

SUBTALAR NEUTRAL STIRRUP ANKLE SUPPORT AND MODIFIED HIGH DYE

Indications

This technique is effective for treating plantar fasciitis, frequent ankle sprains or weak ankles, ankle or foot tendinitis, shin splints, "fallen arches" (pronated feet), tarsal coalition, calcaneal bursitis, and Achilles tendinitis and is also effective for ankle fracture rehabilitation. It is commonly used for clients who perform activities barefoot or in shoes that are tight or offer little support.

Client's Position

The client is prone with the foot hanging off the end of the table; an alternate position is supine with the heel hanging off the table, ankle in 0° dorsiflexion and in subtalar neutral.

Physical Therapist's Position

The PT is sitting on a stool or chair at the end of the table.

Application Guidelines

1. Place a horizontal piece of strapping tape around the ankle at the malleoli as an anchor (if the skin is hairy or sensitive, you can use underwrap first) (a).
2. Place the foot in subtalar neutral and neutral dorsiflexion.
3. Starting at the lateral malleolus anchor strip, pull a piece of tape around the bottom of the foot, just inside the arch (ensuring not to cause skin wrinkles on the plantar aspect of the foot), around the navicular, and up to the medial malleolus, keeping the ankle in neutral (no excessive inversion or eversion). This is a stirrup strip (b-c).
4. Reinforce with a second stirrup strip to better support the arch.
5. This method can also be combined with the arch taping technique for modified high dye (d).

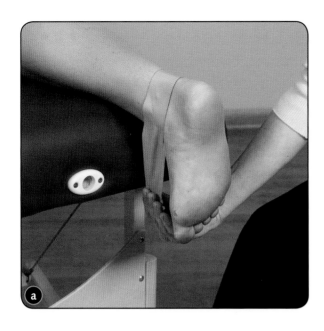

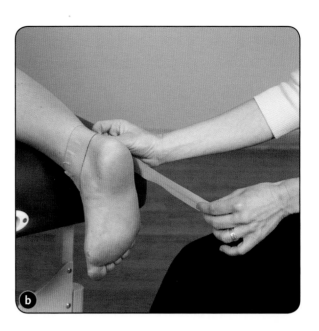

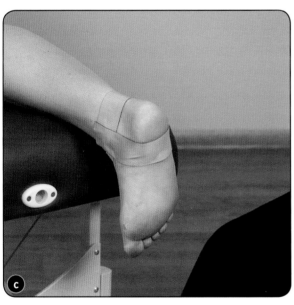

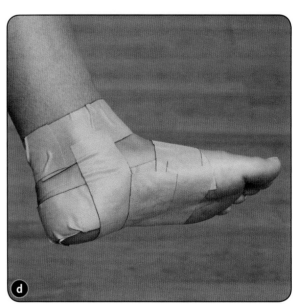

CALCANEUS INVERSION GLIDE

Indications

This technique is effective for treating plantar fasciitis and heel pain.

Client's Position

The client is supine with the leg in external rotation.

Physical Therapist's Position

The PT is sitting or standing, facing the client's foot.

Application Guidelines (Mulligan)

1. Perform a calcaneal inversion glide: Stabilize the client's tibia and fibula with one hand, and invert the calcaneus with the other hand.

2. Starting on the lateral posterior calcaneus (*a*) while maintaining the calcaneal inversion glide (*b*), pull a piece of half-width strapping tape around the heel and across the medial malleolus, anchoring the tape to the lateral lower leg (*c*).

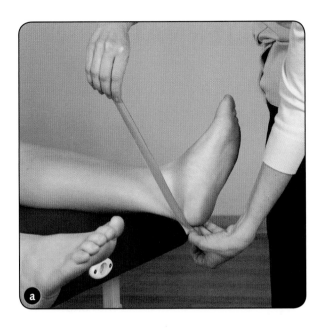

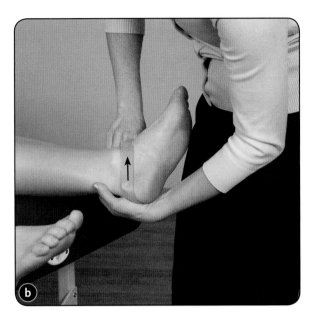

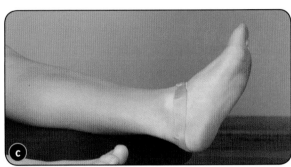

CALCANEUS INVERSION: ALTERNATIVE TECHNIQUE

🔘 **DVD** VIDEO

Indications

This technique is effective for treating plantar fasciitis and heel pain.

Client's Position

The client is supine with the leg in external rotation.

Physical Therapist's Position

The PT is sitting or standing, facing the client's foot.

Application Guidelines (Mulligan)

1. Apply the first piece of tape just distal to the lateral malleolus, pulling the calcaneus medially, and attach the tape to the medial aspect of the foot distal to the medial malleolus (*a-b*).

2. Apply the second and third pieces in the same pattern, with overlap of approximately one-third of the tape width, moving in the distal direction (*c*).

3. Apply the fourth piece of tape around the back of the heel, starting distal to the lateral malleolus, wrapping around the posterior aspect of the calcaneus, and anchoring distal to the medial malleolus (*d-e*); this anchors the first three pieces of tape (Hyland et al. 2006).

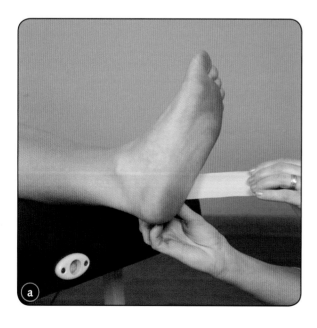

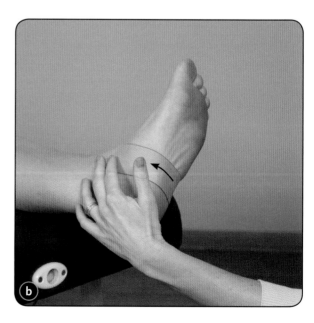

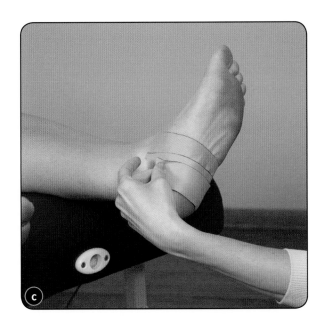

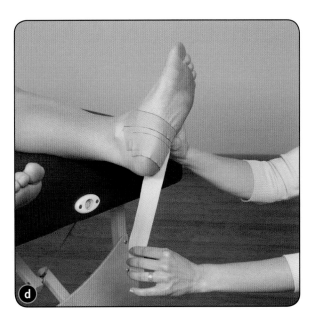

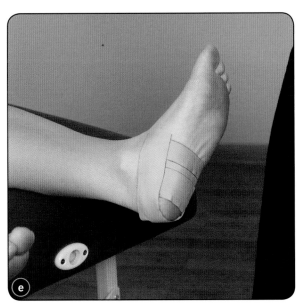

ACHILLES UNLOADING

Indication

This technique is effective for treating Achilles tendinitis or partial tears as well as Sever's disease.

Client's Position

The client is prone with the foot hanging off the end of the table; an alternative position is supine with the heel hanging off the table, ankle in 0° dorsiflexion and in subtalar neutral.

Physical Therapist's Position

The PT is sitting on a stool or chair at the end of the table.

Screen

Perform the Achilles unloading test: Apply compressive force to the Achilles tendon as the patient performs the aggravating activity or rises up on the toes (a).

Application Guidelines

1. If symptoms are relieved, tape a horizontal strip around the malleoli of the ankle (b).

2. Reinforce with one or two pieces of strapping tape. For the Mulligan technique, do not overlap the tape strips (c-d).

3. Performing arch taping and stirrup techniques (see photos a-d of *Subtalar Neutral Stirrup Ankle Support*, pages 26-27) together will often reduce symptoms of Achilles problems.

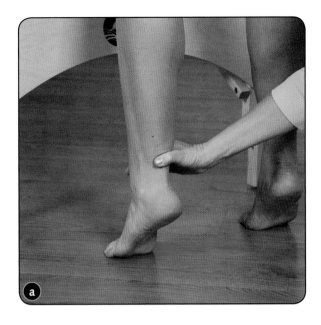

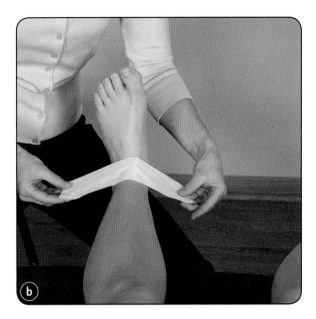

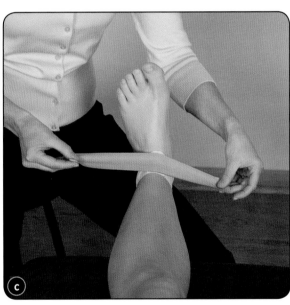

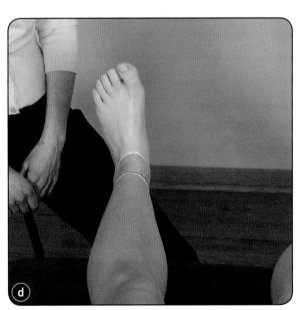

HYPERMOBILE DISTAL FIBULA

Indications

This technique is effective for treating chronic lateral ankle pain, pain in the lateral ankle with dorsiflexion or plantar flexion, and persons with a history of ankle inversion sprains or rolling.

Client's Position

The client is either supine or prone with the foot hanging off the edge of the table.

Physical Therapist's Position

The PT is sitting at the end of the table.

Screen

Perform the fibular glide assessment: The patient is supine, with the fibula mobilized anteriorly and posteriorly (a); the test is positive if pain is elicited or the displacement of the fibula is greater than on the uninvolved side (Beumer et al. 2002).

Application Guidelines (Mulligan)

1. Have the patient perform the aggravating activity while you manually glide the distal fibula anteriorly or posteriorly, whichever position eases the symptoms.

2. Place 3 to 6 inches (7.5 to 15 cm) of underwrap horizontally over the distal fibula (b).

3. Apply strapping tape, starting anterior to the distal fibula and pulling posteriorly with overpressure to glide the fibula; anchor the tape to the posterior leg (c-d). Do not completely encircle the ankle. Less common is placing the fibula in posterior glide to decrease symptoms or starting posteriorly and pulling anteriorly if anterior glide decreases symptoms, using one or two pieces of strapping tape to reinforce.

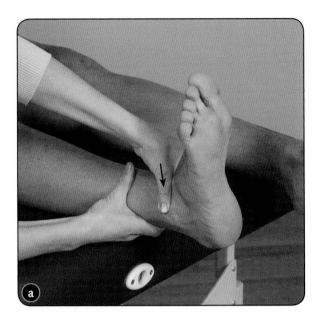

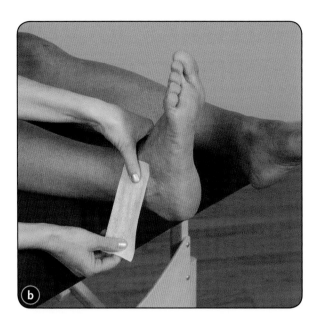

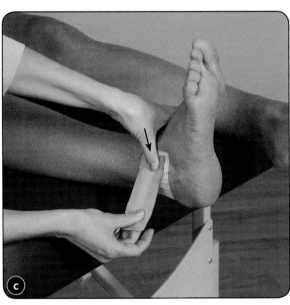

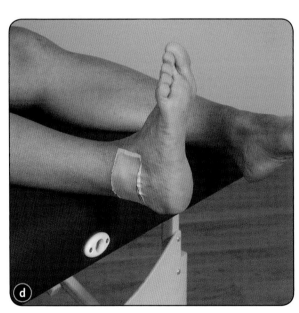

HALLUX ABDUCTOVALGUS (HAV) BUNION CORRECTION

Indications

This technique is effective for treating MTP joint sprains, plantar ligament injuries (hyperflexion), turf toe (LCL hyperextension injury), and bunions at the first MTP joint.

Client's Position

The client is supine with the foot hanging off the edge of the table.

Physical Therapist's Position

The PT is sitting at the end of the table.

Application Guidelines

1. Start the strapping tape distal to the interphalangeal (IP) joint of the first toe (*a*).
2. While applying some force to abduct the toe, pull tape around to the fifth metatarsal, without causing too much discomfort (*b*).
3. Apply anchor strips distal to the MTP joints and around first toe (*c-d*).

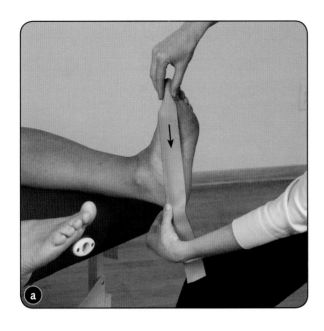

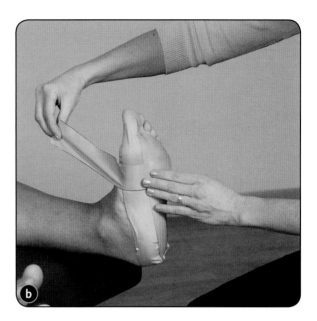

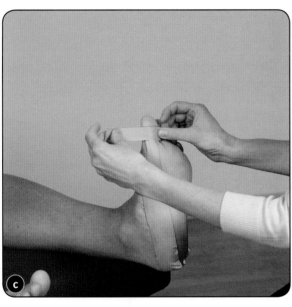

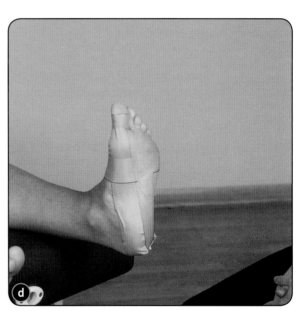

FIRST METATARSAL–CUNEIFORM GLIDE

Indication

This technique is effective for treating midfoot pain and medial foot pain or volar or plantar pain at the cuneiform with inversion.

Client's Position

The client is supine with the foot hanging off the end of the table.

Physical Therapist's Position

The PT is standing or sitting at the end of the table, facing the client's foot. A second clinician may be required to assist with taping.

Screen

Perform a first metatarsal–cuneiform glide (a): If pain is reported at the top or medial foot, joint mobility of the first metatarsal–cuneiform joint could be impaired. A medial glide to the first metatarsal (MT) combined with a lateral glide of the cuneiform decreases symptoms in this area of the foot.

Application Guidelines (Mulligan)

1. Place a strip of half-width strapping tape at the medial foot, and pull superiorly while applying overpressure to the cuneiform (b-c).

2. Apply a plantar glide to the first metatarsal. Start the half-width strapping tape here, pulling it around the plantar foot to the lateral side of the foot (d-e).

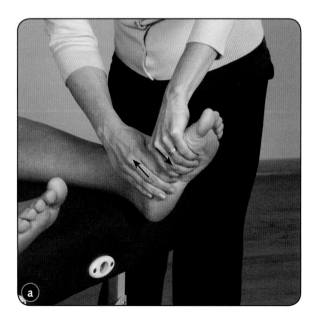

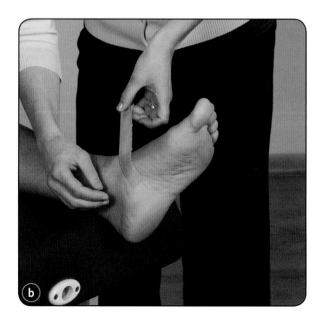

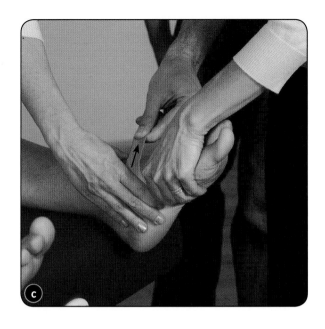

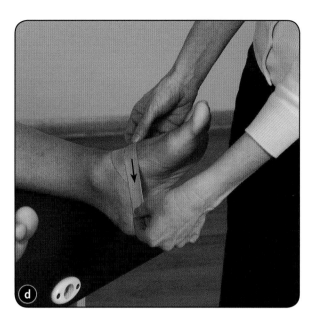

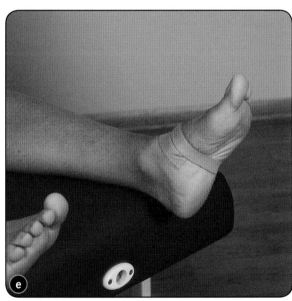

FIFTH METATARSAL DORSAL GLIDE

Indication

This technique elevates the fifth MT, fourth MT, or both to relieve lateral foot pain.

Client's Position

The client is supine.

Physical Therapist's Position

The PT is standing, facing the client's foot. A second clinician may be required to assist with taping.

Screen

Perform a fifth metatarsal dorsal glide (Mulligan): Elevate the fifth or fourth metatarsal, or both, for relief of lateral foot pain (*a*).

Application Guidelines (Mulligan)

1. Apply plantar-to-dorsal force to the fourth or fifth proximal metatarsal, or both.
2. Start the half-width strapping tape on the plantar lateral foot, pulling the tape over the top of the foot and anchoring it on the medial ankle (*b-c*).

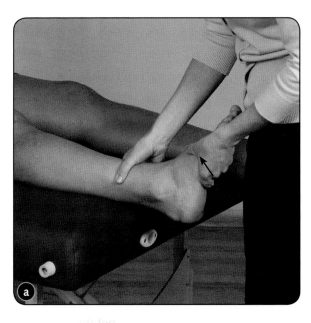

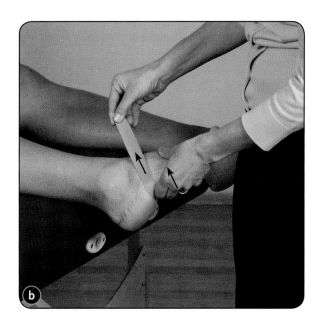

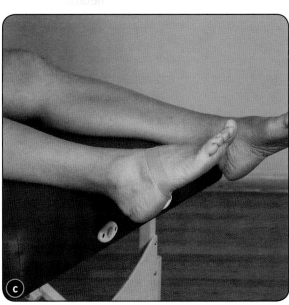

FIFTH METATARSAL–CUBOID DORSAL AND PLANTAR GLIDE

Indication

This technique is effective for treating pain over the cuboid on the lateral foot, a common injury in snowboarding.

Client's Position

The client is supine.

Physical Therapist's Position

The PT is facing the client's foot. A second clinician may be required to assist with taping.

Screen

To ease pain over the cuboid, perform a lateral glide between the cuboid and the fifth metatarsal. Locate the styloid process of the fifth MT. Stabilize the fifth MT, and apply a superior (dorsal) glide to the cuboid for pain relief.

Application Guidelines (Mulligan)

1. Place half-width strapping tape on the plantar lateral foot at the cuboid, applying force superiorly (*a*).

2. Place a second piece of tape on top of the lateral foot at the fifth MT, and glide in the opposite direction (plantarly). Anchor the tape on the medial foot (*b-c*).

3. The glides can be reversed if a plantar glide of the cuboid and a superior glide of the fifth MT relieve symptoms (opposing tape forces). Strips should not cross the cuboid–MT joint line and should not overlap.

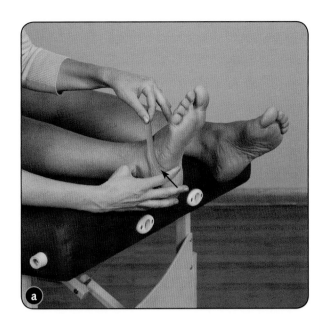

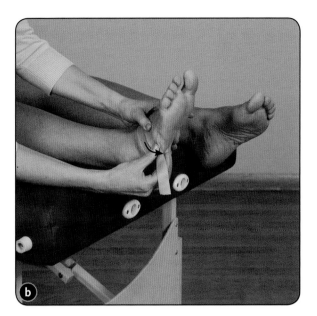

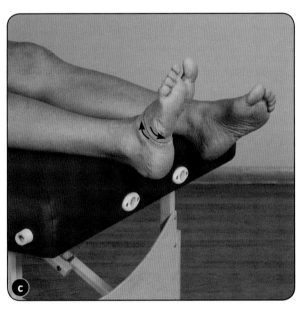

GASTROCNEMIUS UNLOADING

Indications

This technique is effective for treating Achilles tendinitis or gastrocnemius pain as well as pain decreased with lateral glide in either area.

Client's Position

The client is prone.

Physical Therapist's Position

The PT is standing, facing the client's leg.

Screen

If pain is present in either head of the gastrocnemius, perform a gastrocnemius unloading test by applying a compressive or medial or lateral force to the muscle while the client performs the aggravating activity (*a*). A reduction in pain indicates this taping technique will be beneficial.

Application Guidelines (Mulligan)

1. Apply underwrap to the affected head of the gastrocnemius (*b*).

2. Follow with strapping tape, pulling medially or laterally (depending on which direction decreased symptoms) and gliding the tendon or muscle belly (*c*); anchor the tape around the anterior shin (*d*).

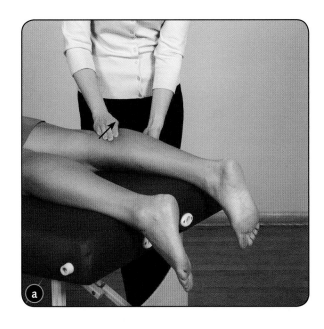

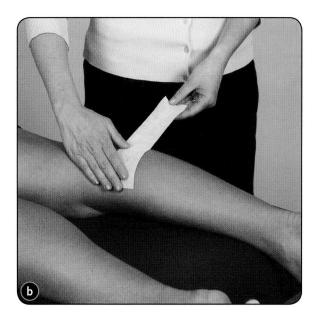

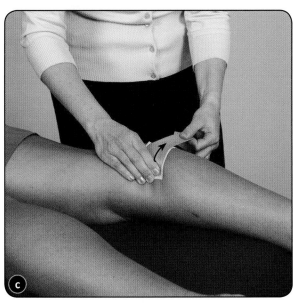

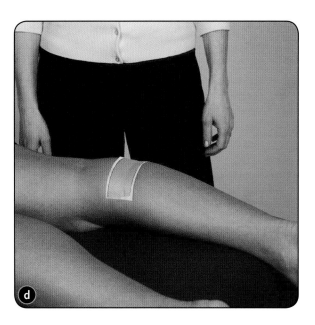

BRACES

The following braces simulate taping techniques:

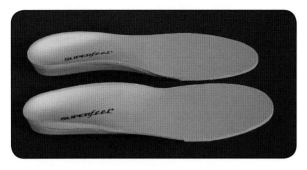

Off-the-shelf orthotics (e.g., Superfeet): Inexpensive full-foot shoe inserts are available for clients who do not want to purchase expensive custom orthotics. Off-the-shelf orthotics provide minimal arch support and good cushioning, and they last approximately 18 months depending on activity.

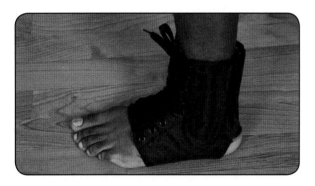

Ankle support (lace-up): Elastic or lace-up over-the-counter ankle supports are used to control edema and to increase stability or proprioception.

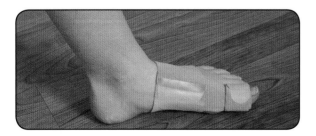

HAV (bunion) corrector: This bulky over-the-counter brace may help correct the position of the first toe. It is used at night when not bearing weight on the foot.

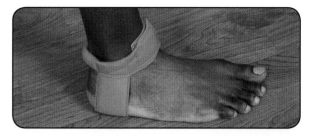

Achilles tendon strap (e.g., Cho-Pat): Found in some medical supply stores, these straps are an alternative to Achilles tendon taping for the treatment of chronic Achilles tendinitis.

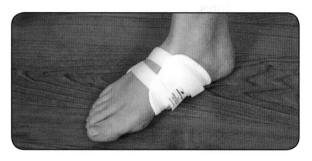

Arch-lifter brace: This bulky over-the-counter brace may provide support but cannot be worn in all shoes or for certain activities. I have not found this brace effective.

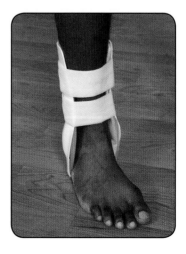

Ankle immobilizer brace (e.g., Aircast): Over-the-counter braces are used for ankle instability, ligament laxity, or decreased tolerance to full weight bearing. They are bulky and cannot be worn with all shoes.

Custom orthotics (e.g., Sole Supports): These total-contact orthotics are commonly used by people with pronated feet or chronic arch and heel pain; people who are on their feet for extended periods; and people who perform running, jumping, and impact activities. They come in three-quarter length, full-foot, and low-profile models depending on the activity and the shoe used.

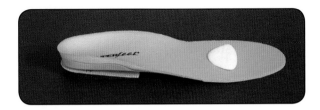

Heel lift: Heel lifts can be found at some medical supply stores. They are used to correct leg length discrepancy and to relieve Achilles tendinitis pain or gastrocnemius strain. Long-term use is not recommended unless advised by a medical professional.

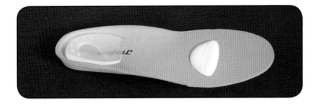

Cutouts and pads: Metatarsal bars, metatarsal pads, and heel spur cutouts are over-the-counter pads used to correct or offload the metatarsals, calcaneal spurs, or other deformities or pains in the foot. The pads can be adhered to inserts or incorporated permanently into custom orthotics.

CASE STUDIES

Taping and lateral ankle pain.

A 20-year-old female sustained an inversion ankle sprain during a fall off a step 2 months ago and reported a constant ache in the anterior and lateral ankle, worse with plantar flexion activities (going up stairs, rising on toes). The X-rays were negative. Exam revealed mild edema at the anterolateral malleolus and a normal gait pattern. She had pain with passive range of motion greater than 15%, a hypermobile distal fibula, and pain with resisted plantar flexion and eversion. In physical therapy, she was given strengthening exercises and range of motion exercises. On her third visit, she rated the pain at 0 to 4 out of 10; this decreased to no pain when the distal fibula was glided anteriorly during ankle plantar flexion, so the ankle was taped in that position. The patient was told to return to therapy only if she had continued problems. She did not return.

Taping and plantar fasciitis.

A 32-year-old female complained of bilateral heel pain with prolonged walking or after being on her feet all day in work shoes or after about 6 miles (10 km) in hiking shoes. Exam showed tight gastrocnemius and soleus and a longer right leg. Patient was given calf stretches, and tape was applied (arch plus stirrup). She brought hiking and work shoes in to the clinic. Work shoes were typical unsupportive ladies dress flats. Hiking shoes were supportive. She reported no pain when taped while wearing work shoes and less pain when taped while wearing hiking shoes. She was instructed to find more supportive work shoes that would eliminate heel pain. She was casted for orthotics for her hiking shoes and advised to wear a left heel lift plus orthotics if the heel was still bothersome. A few months later, she reportedly was able to hike 16 miles (26 km) without heel pain using orthotics.

The Knee

Taping for patellofemoral symptoms (i.e., McConnell taping) is probably the most common use of strap taping at the knee. Taping is very effective in this area because the patella is such a superficial bone, and taping forces can direct the patella's wide range of mobility as it tracks when the quadriceps contract. Many other structures around the knee are also superficial (tendons, fat pads, bursae) and respond well to taping, which is used to offload painful structures.

The following techniques are covered in this chapter: patellar medial glide, patellar tendon unloading, infrapatellar fat pad unloading, pes anserinus bursa unloading, ITB friction syndrome unloading, proximal fibular glide, tibiofemoral torsion, knee hyperextension or varus/valgus blocking, tensor fascia latae (TFL) and hip unloading, and medial hamstring unloading. Also, the subtalar neutral ankle taping and arch taping techniques from chapter 2 (pages 20-26) can be useful for treating knee issues.

Treatments are described for the following problems: patellofemoral syndrome or maltracking (anterior knee pain), dislocating or subluxing patella, patellar tendinitis (jumper's knee), pes anserinus bursitis (medial knee pain), iliotibial band (ITB) friction syndrome (lateral knee pain), plica irritation (medial femoral condyle pain), Osgood-Schlatter disease, bipartite patella, fat pad irritation (infrapatellar pain), pain at the proximal fibular head, tibiofemoral torsion, muscle strains, and knee hyperextension. Use of heel lifts is also discussed.

ANATOMY OF THE KNEE

The distal femur, proximal tibia and fibula, and patella are the bones of the knee. Other ana-tomical entities to consider are the menisci, ligaments, musculotendinous lengths, bursae, synovial plicae, and fat pads. The knee is especially susceptible to injury during twisting, lateral or medial trauma, or hyperextension (ligamentous, meniscal, or patellofemoral injuries), especially when the foot is planted. In activities or sports that involve repetitive motions (e.g., running), overuse injuries can occur. Foot position (especially a pronated foot) can alter neutral anatomical knee position. Anatomical genu varus, genu valgus, or tibial rotation can also predispose a person to certain injuries, especially if the muscle strength is not balanced around the knee, hip, and lumbopelvic region.

EVIDENCE

Taping and patellofemoral pain syndrome (PFPS). Patellar taping was originally developed by Jenny McConnell, PT, as an adjunct to the treatment for PFPS. Since then, patellar taping has gained widespread acceptance in the treatment of this condition and others (Crossley et al. 2000) and has been widely studied compared with other taping techniques for the knee.

The evidence to support interventions in the management of PFPS is growing. Physical therapy treatments that include taping have been shown to consistently improve short-term pain and function (Crossley et al. 2001; Herrington and Payton 1997; Christou 2004; Whittingham, Palmer, and MacMillan 2004). In a study by Crossley et al. (2002), taping corrections were applied in the order of anterior tilt, medial tilt, glide, and fat pad unloading until the participant's pain was reduced by at least 50%. Wilson et al. (2003) found that patellar taping produced an immediate decrease in pain in patients with

49

Anterior Knee

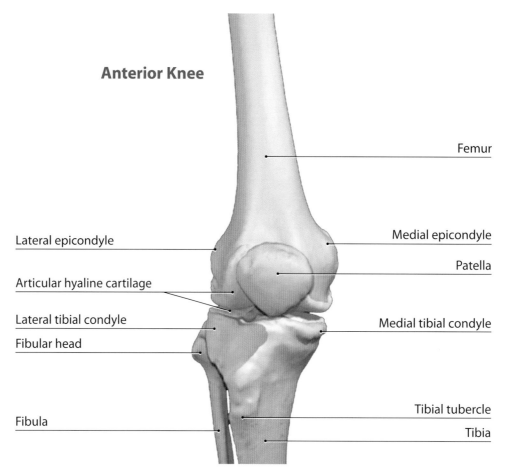

Femur

Medial epicondyle

Lateral epicondyle

Patella

Articular hyaline cartilage

Lateral tibial condyle

Medial tibial condyle

Fibular head

Tibial tubercle

Fibula

Tibia

Image courtesy of Primal Pictures.

Posterior Knee

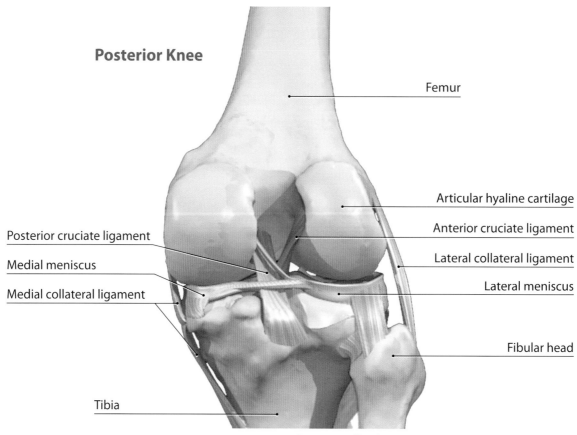

Femur

Articular hyaline cartilage

Anterior cruciate ligament

Posterior cruciate ligament

Lateral collateral ligament

Medial meniscus

Lateral meniscus

Medial collateral ligament

Fibular head

Tibia

Image courtesy of Primal Pictures.

Anterior Thigh Muscles

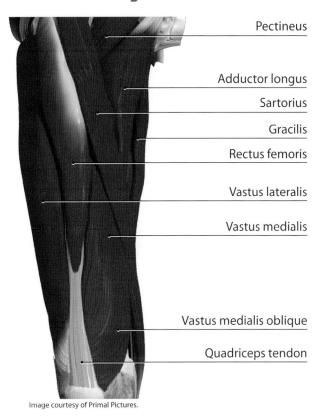

Pectineus

Adductor longus

Sartorius

Gracilis

Rectus femoris

Vastus lateralis

Vastus medialis

Vastus medialis oblique

Quadriceps tendon

Image courtesy of Primal Pictures.

Posterior Thigh Muscles

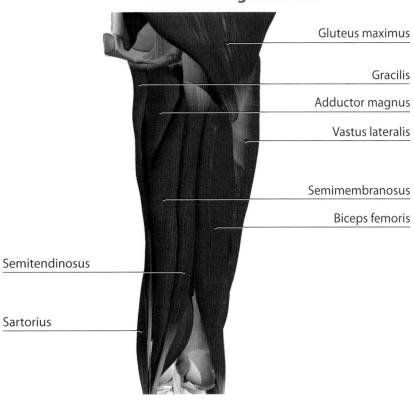

Gluteus maximus

Gracilis

Adductor magnus

Vastus lateralis

Semimembranosus

Biceps femoris

Semitendinosus

Sartorius

Image courtesy of Primal Pictures.

Surface Anatomy, Posterier Knee

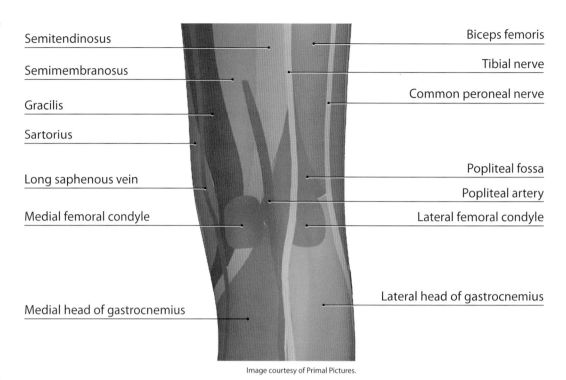

Semitendinosus

Semimembranosus

Gracilis

Sartorius

Long saphenous vein

Medial femoral condyle

Medial head of gastrocnemius

Biceps femoris

Tibial nerve

Common peroneal nerve

Popliteal fossa

Popliteal artery

Lateral femoral condyle

Lateral head of gastrocnemius

Image courtesy of Primal Pictures.

Surface Anatomy, Anterior Knee

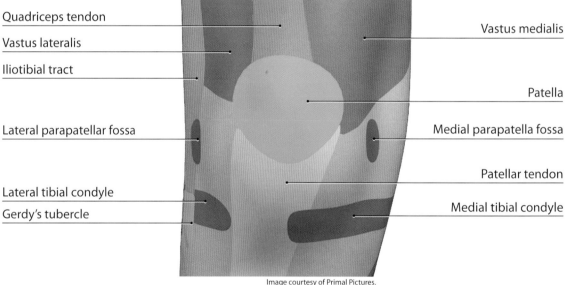

Quadriceps tendon

Vastus lateralis

Iliotibial tract

Lateral parapatellar fossa

Lateral tibial condyle

Gerdy's tubercle

Vastus medialis

Patella

Medial parapatella fossa

Patellar tendon

Medial tibial condyle

Image courtesy of Primal Pictures.

PFPS, regardless of which taping technique was used.

Interventions for PFPS include a combination of the following:

- Patellar taping
- Bracing
- Strengthening the vastus medialis obliquus and other muscles surrounding the knee and hip
- Iliotibial band stretching
- Using orthotics

PFPS can be caused by direct trauma to the knee, or the cause can be insidious. Altered lower extremity biomechanics such as poor hip rotation control, excessive foot pronation, femoral anteversion, tibial torsion, or tight muscles are thought to contribute to PFPS by altering patellofemoral kinematics. Patellar displacement with taping partially explains the previously documented decrease in pain caused by increases in patellofemoral contact area (Derasari et al. 2010).

The characteristics of patients with PFPS who respond favorably to a specific patellar taping technique were identified, and Hyland et al. (2006) developed a clinical prediction rule (CPR) incorporating the findings. Patients who present with tibial varum greater than 5° or a positive patellar tilt test responded favorably with medial glide patellar taping. The results of this study indicate that patients with PFPS who have one of the two characteristics identified in the CPR may benefit from patellar taping with a medial glide component as an initial treatment.

Randomized or quasi-randomized studies assessing patellar taping or bracing effects on chronic knee pain from seven electronic databases (to November 2006) investigated patellar taping or bracing effects in people with anterior knee pain as well as taping effects in people with knee osteoarthritis (OA). Evidence suggests that taping applied with a medially directed force on the patella produces a clinically meaningful change in chronic knee pain. There was limited evidence demonstrating the efficacy of patellar bracing (Warden et al. 2008).

Taping and quadriceps or muscle function. Gilleard, McConnell, and Parsons (1998) found that when the patellofemoral joint was taped, the vastus medialis oblique (VMO) was activated earlier than the vastus lateralis (VL) during step-up and step-down tasks. Patellar taping compared with no tape may improve knee extensor strength during weight-bearing activities such as the lateral step-up exercise and the vertical jump (Ernst, Kawaguchi, and Saliba 1999). Conversely, a study by Ng and Cheng (2002) noted a decrease in relative activity of the VMO after taping, implying that it may not be suitable to combine patellar taping with VMO facilitative exercise training.

Research into the effect of patellar taping in asymptomatic persons shows conflicting results. When studies had positive findings, these effects appear to be negated by exercise. Herrington's study (2009) found that patellar position was significantly changed after the application of tape. Although low-intensity exercise resulted in a significant change in patellar position compared with the taped position before exercise, that change most likely occurred because of chance or measurement error. Patellar taping had a detrimental effect on normal quadriceps function (Herrington 2004), possibly due to a subtle alteration in the alignment of the extensor mechanism, causing it to function less optimally. This research supports the hypothesis that taping may alter patellar position and with it the efficient functioning of the extensor mechanism.

The effects of patellar taping on quadriceps peak torque and perceived pain levels of PFPS patients were studied during maximal quadriceps contractions (Herrington 2001). In all subjects, patellar taping reduced perceived pain levels and improved peak torque during both eccentric and concentric contraction and at both testing velocities. The results show that taping of the patella provides a useful adjunct to treatment, especially if the goal of treatment is improvement in quadriceps strength.

Taping and muscle inhibition. Firm taping across the VL muscle belly in asymptomatic patients significantly decreases VL activity during stair descent (Tobin and Robinson 2000). The tape could change the orientation of the fascia or could simply have a proprioceptive effect, influencing pain; Hall et al. 1995). Taping on the posterior thigh could inhibit an overactive hamstring muscle, which is a protective response to mechanical provocation of neural tissue (Hall et al. 1995).

Patellar taping reduces anterior knee pain during the mini-squat in people with patellofemoral pain and patellofemoral joint malalignment, but it cannot facilitate vastus medialis obliquus activity (Ng and Cheng 2002).

Taping and proprioception. In a study by Callaghan et al. (2008), patellar taping did not improve proprioception in patients with PFPS, but a subgroup of PFPS patients with poor proprioception may exist and be helped by patellar taping.

Taping and patellofemoral joint OA. Knee taping is a beneficial treatment for the management of pain and disability in patients with knee osteoarthritis (Hinman et al. 2003).

In a study by Crossley et al. (2009), patients with patellofemoral OA showed greater lateral patellar displacement and bisect offset compared with controls. In the patellofemoral joint OA group, patellar taping resulted in a significant decrease in lateral alignment, with reduced lateral displacement and increased lateral patellar tilt angle. Pain during squatting decreased when patients were taped, indicating that patellar taping may reduce malalignment and pain associated with patellofemoral joint OA.

Patients with symptomatic OA of the knee are advised to use patellar taping for short-term relief of pain and improvement in function. This recommendation is addressed by a level II systematic review examining the use of patellar taping among patients with symptomatic OA of the knee. The randomized controlled trials (RCTs) in the systematic review report statistically significant and possibly clinically important effects of medial taping on pain immediately and 4 days after the start of taping. This effect is observed only when taping is compared with no taping, not when medial taping is compared with sham taping (Richmond et al. 2009).

In a randomized controlled trial of a physical therapy–based intervention for patellofemoral joint OA, the treatment group had a small decrease in pain and a significant increase in quadriceps strength of the knee. After 1 year there were no significant differences in any outcome measure (Quilty et al. 2003). Patellar taping is a simple, safe, economical way of providing short-term pain relief in patients with osteoarthritis of the patellofemoral joint (Cushnaghan, McCarthy, and Dieppe 1994). In this study, medial taping of the patella was significantly better than the neutral or lateral taping for pain scores, symptom change, and patient preference. The tape resulted in a 25% reduction in knee pain.

EVALUATION

Perform a thorough history, evaluation and strength test including the back, abdominals and core, hip, and lower leg. Review all tests (e.g., X-rays) to help determine the appropriate taping method. Table 3.1 provides the normal active range of motion (AROM) of the knee.

TABLE 3.1

Normal AROM of Knee

Motion	Degree
Knee flexion	135°
Knee extension	0-15°
Medial tibial rotation on femur	20-30°
Lateral tibial rotation on femur	30-40°

Adapted from Magee 2006

Special Tests

Testing for patellar tracking and alignment, joint instability and internal derangement, and performing the Plica test are discussed in the following sections.

Patellar Position and Tracking

Assess for patellar tracking and alignment with the patient supine. Palpate the superior poles of the patella while the client's leg is relaxed. Maintaining contact with the superior patella, have the client contract the quadriceps muscle and note which direction your fingers over the poles travel up the thigh. Evaluate the following components of alignment: medial and lateral glide, medial and lateral displacement, medial and lateral tilt, anterior tilt, and rotation. Despite the low reliability of this assessment procedure for patellofemoral positioning, physical therapists use it often.

Medial and lateral displacement are assessed by observing and comparing the distance between the midpoint of the patella to the medial and lateral femoral epicondyles. The distance should be fairly equal. If the patella is displaced laterally, the distance on the lateral side is smaller. Medial and lateral tilt are assessed by comparing the height of the two borders of the patella on the transverse plane. If the lateral border is more pronounced, it indicates a lateral tilt.

Anterior tilt is determined by palpating the inferior pole of the patella; if no significant anterior tilt exists, the inferior pole should be easily palpated (Fitzgerald and McClure1995). Rotation is assessed by examining the orientation of the long axis of the patella with that of the femur, which should normally be in line with the anterior superior iliac spine (ASIS). If the distal end of the longitudinal axis of the patella is lateral to the ASIS, then the patella is considered to be rotated laterally. If the axis is more medial, it is medially rotated.

To assess patellar tracking, as stated above, palpate the superior poles of the patella, and ask the patient to contract the quadriceps muscles while compressing the popliteal fossa against the examining table (see figure *a* on page 59. Note how much patellar movement is present and how the patella tracks. Ideally, the patella should follow the midline of the femur but often tracks laterally to the midline, indicating a possible imbalance in the quadriceps musculature. Compare with the uninvolved knee. As a screening test, if pain is present in the anterior knee on stairs, apply medial pressure to the lateral edge of the patella as the patient ascends stairs. If this decreases patellar pain, patellar medial glide correction may be a helpful technique.

Joint Instability and Internal Derangement

Ruling out ligamentous laxity and joint or meniscal issues is essential by performing the Lachman test or anterior drawer test for anterior cruciate ligament (ACL) laxity, performing the valgus and varus stress test for medial and lateral collateral ligament (MCL and LCL) laxity, and performing the McMurray test or assessing joint-line tenderness for meniscal problems. Refer to Cleland 2007 for details.

Plica Test

Meniscal symptoms can mimic plica irritation (Hertling and Kessler 1996). To assess for plica irritation in supine, apply medial patellar pressure and medial tibial rotation while the knee is flexed and extended between 30 and 90°. Normally the medial patellar plica is involved if the symptoms of anteromedial knee pain occur, possibly with a snapping sensation as the thickened, inflamed plica snaps over the medial femoral condyle. Often the plica is tender and inflamed on the anteromedial knee as compared with the other leg (Magee 2006).

Biomechanical Considerations

Knee position, foot pronation, pelvic control and strength as well as hip strength, and leg length discrepancy are important biomechanical considerations. These considerations and related assessments are discussed in the following section.

Knee Position: Varus, Valgus, and Quadriceps (Q) Angle

The Q angle is measured by lines drawn (or estimated) from the center of the patella to the anterior superior iliac spine (ASIS) and to the center of the tibial tuberosity (figure 3.1). An angle of 10 to 15° is normal. The larger the Q angle, the more lateral the pull on the patella. Patients with valgus (or "knock") knees have increased Q angles. Varus knees ("bowlegged") can exhibit decreased Q angle. The Q angle can be affected by foot position (the angle tends to increase with increased foot pronation) (Grelsamer and McConnell 1998).

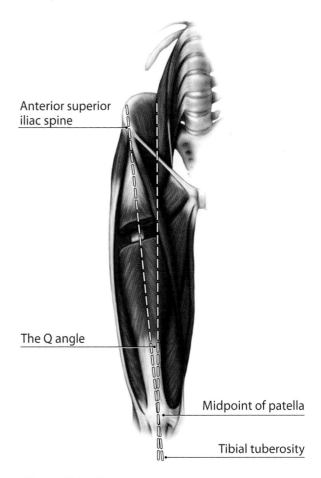

Anterior superior iliac spine

The Q angle

Midpoint of patella

Tibial tuberosity

Figure 3.1   Q angle.
Reprinted from R. Behnke, 2005, *Kinetic anatomy*, 2nd ed. (Champaign, IL: Human Kinetics), 200.

Pronated Foot Correction

Assess foot position and navicular drop in standing position. Have the patient supinate the foot to increase the arch space while keeping the metatarsal heads on the floor. Have the patient ascend a stair in this corrected position. If anterior knee pain is decreased or there is a significant difference between arch space with the foot relaxed and supinated, then taping for subtalar neutral and arch support may be helpful. This can be done in addition to or instead of taping the patella, depending on the results of the evaluation.

Single-Leg Step-Down Biomechanical Assessment

To ensure adequate pelvic control and strength as well as hip strength, assess the biomechanics of the lower extremity while the patient simulates required activities. First, observe the patient's gait pattern for any orthopedic or neurological deviations in neutral leg position or muscle control. The majority of the time, this will appear normal. Next, ask the patient to stand on one leg; note if the pelvis remains level (i.e., the iliac crests stay parallel to the floor, and one hip does not drop with the shift of weight). A progression to a step-up or step-down on a stair is important to observe for anatomical limb alignment (i.e., the foot is not overpronated, the knee is not excessively internally or externally rotated, the legs remain parallel, and the hips remain even).

Leg Length Discrepancy

A leg length discrepancy can be tested multiple ways. Typically start with the patient in standing; check iliac crest height symmetry, both visually and by palpation. With the patient prone, first palpate iliac crest and ischial tuberosity to check the length of each ilia, then from greater trochanter to fibular head to check femur length (or compare knee height in supine hook-lying position). Ask the patient to bend his knees, and visually check tibial length bilaterally (prone knee flexion test for tibial shortening). Identify where the length discrepancy is in the lower half. A heel lift may be indicated in the shoe of the shorter leg, depending on severity (Magee 2006). See chapter 2, pages 18 and 19.

Hypermobile Joint Protection

If the patient has genu recurvatum (knee hyperextension in standing, found in many athletes for whom flexibility is advantageous, such as dancers and gymnasts), this joint hypermobility needs to be addressed. Advise the patient to refrain from locking the knees during certain activities and to engage the quadriceps muscles and maintain slight knee flexion while at rest in order to protect the joint and minimize pressure on the patella. Joint hypermobility accompanied by symptoms such as pain or repetitive joint sprains is termed joint hypermobility syndrome (JHS). JHS is an underrecognized and poorly managed systemic and hereditary connective tissue disorder, resulting in repeated intermittent pain or injuries of multiple joint areas. It is more prevalent in females, and symptoms often start in childhood and continue into adulthood. Management includes education in behavior modification for activities; physical therapy including manual therapy, taping and bracing, and other modalities; and collaboration with other medical professionals. Progress is often slow, but with a specifically designed management strategy, a decrease in symptoms and functional fitness can be attained (Simmonds and Keer 2007).

Heel Lifts

There are two schools of thought about heel lifts: One recommends them, one does not. There is no consensus in the literature about the effects of leg length discrepancies (LLDs) and the best interventions for treating them. Following are some important factors to consider before suggesting a heel lift: whether the leg length discrepancy is anatomical (bone has asymmetrical length compared to other side) or functional (if the body accommodated to the difference and there are no symptoms, there is no need to use a heel lift); the age of the client (heel lifts are typically more effective in a younger population because older clients may have accommodated to the discrepancy, and adding a lift may cause problems elsewhere in the body); the client's level of activity (more active persons may benefit more from a heel lift); the accuracy of the method used to measure the discrepancy; height difference between legs (the larger the difference, the more helpful the lift might be); and possible improvement in or worsening of pain or symptoms in the low back, hip, knee, ankle, and gait kinematics.

A length difference of between 3 and 20 mm is clinically significant. A 3 mm difference may require intervention for higher-level athletes such as runners (Subotnick 1981) or dancers. Runners may be more sensitive to smaller discrepancies and more prone to injuries. A 6 mm difference in runners may equal a 19 mm difference in the general population (Subotnick 1981) because of increased weight-bearing forces on the heel during running. A difference of 9 mm would be sufficient to cause low back pain (Giles and Taylor 1981) in the general population. A 20 mm discrepancy could produce impairment (Lampe, Swierstra, and Diepstraten 1996).

Effects on gait: Discrepancies between 20 and 30 mm were found to increase ground reaction forces and energy expenditure of the lower extremity (Kaufmann, Miller, and Sutherland 1996). Heel lifts equalized the difference in cadence between the longer and shorter leg. Compensatory pronation in the longer leg and supination in the shorter leg were corrected with a lift (D'Amico, Dinowitz, and Polchaninoff 1985). After correction to within 10 mm, the ground reaction forces were equal in both legs, and stance times were also equalized (Bhave, Paley, and Herzenberg 1999).

There is no specific protocol regarding when to use heel lifts. It should be determined on a case by case basis for differences of less than 5 mm in runners (Gross 1983) and dancers. Heel lift use in dancers with a 2 mm LLD significantly decreased chronic low back pain. In patients aged 17 to 39 with low back pain, scoliosis due to LLD can be improved or corrected with a lift (Giles and Taylor 1981; Papaioannou, Stokes, and Kenwright 1982); in one study, 73% of patients with LBP and a LLD between 8 and 12 mm were symptom free after using a lift (Friberg et al. 1983).

Inside-shoe heel lifts vs. platform (on sole of shoe) lifts: Corrections are recommended externally (on the sole of the shoe) for differences of greater than 10 mm (Gross 2003) to prevent unnecessary Achilles tendon shortening or an increase in lumbar lordosis (Defrin et al. 2005). The use of platform lifts significantly reduced LBP intensity and disability scores.

Recommended wearing schedule: Increase platform lifts no more than 3 to 6 mm at a time, and do not correct for more than half the discrepancy, making adjustments every 2 weeks until desired correction is attained (Blustein and D'Amico 1985).

Technique	Screening tool
Patellar gliding	Patellar position and glide assessment
Patellar tendon unloading	Patellar tendon unloading test
Infrapatellar fat pad unloading	Fat pad unloading test
Pes bursa unloading	Pes bursa unloading test
ITB tendon unloading	ITB unloading test
Proximal fibular glide	Accessory tibiofibular joint testing
TFL unloading	TFL glide
Medial hamstring unloading	Medial hamstring glide

Foot position should be evaluated for all.

PATELLAR MEDIAL GLIDE (PLUS TILT CORRECTIONS)

Indications

This technique is effective for treating dislocating or subluxing patella, patellofemoral syndrome, anterior knee pain, patellar tendinitis, plica irritation, and bipartite patella.

Client's Position

The client is long sitting on a table, with a rolled towel or small bolster under the knee.

Physical Therapist's Position

The PT is standing, facing the affected leg.

Screen

Patellar tracking assessment (a).

Application Guidelines (McConnell)

1. First correct the worst problem with patellar tracking, and then reassess for symptom improvement before applying subsequent techniques to the knee. A 5 mm lateral patellar displacement is significant. The goal is at least a 50% decrease in symptoms with taping (Grelsamer and McConnell 1998).

2. Start by applying a piece of underwrap, approximately 5 to 6 inches (13 to 15 cm) long, over the patella or with the lower edge of the tape bisecting the patella horizontally.

3. Place strapping tape on the lateral patellar border, apply a medial glide to the patella, and pull the tape medially toward the medial hamstring tendons. The underwrap will wrinkle under the strapping tape (b).

4. Reinforce with a second piece of tape (c). To help anchor this, a piece of underwrap can be cut for each edge of the tape and placed vertically to keep the edges from peeling off.

5. To correct for anterior or posterior patellar tilt, place the tape on the superior aspect of the patella to tip the patella out of the fat pad; tape as outlined previously.

6. To correct for lateral patellar tilt, place the tape in the center of the patella and pull medially toward the hamstring tendons (d). Pull laterally to correct medial tilt.

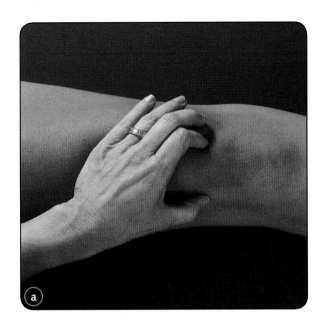

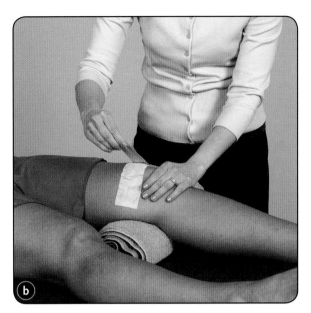

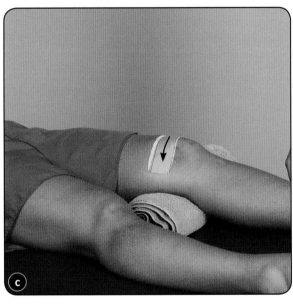

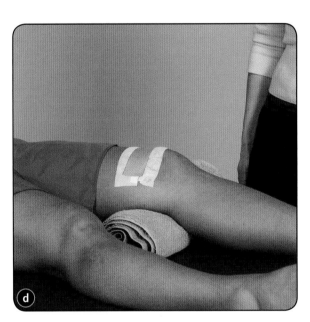

PATELLAR TENDON UNLOADING

Indications

This technique is effective for treating patellofemoral syndrome, patellar tendinitis (jumper's knee), and Osgood-Schlatter disease.

Client's Position

The client is long sitting on a table, with a rolled towel or small bolster under the knee maintaining about 30 degrees of flexion.

Physical Therapist's Position

The PT is standing, facing the affected leg.

Screen

Perform the patellar tendon unloading test (*a*): If pain is present in the anterior knee or patellar tendon with stairs, apply posterior pressure to the patellar tendon as the patient ascends stairs. If this decreases peripatellar pain, the patellar tendon unloading or fat pad unloading technique may be helpful.

Application Guidelines

1. Follow the McConnell taping sequence for medial patellar glide, but place the tape inferior to the patellar.
2. Start with an underwrap strip, approximately 6 inches (15 cm) long, across the patellar tendon, with the knee at around 30° flexion (*b*).
3. Apply strapping tape with a medial pull starting at the lateral edge of the underwrap (*c*). The underwrap will wrinkle under the strapping tape.
4. Reinforce with another strip of tape (*d*).

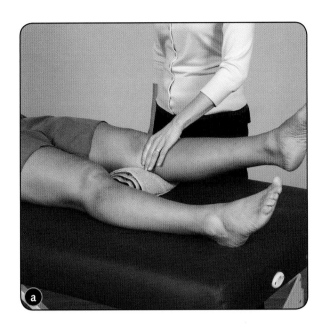

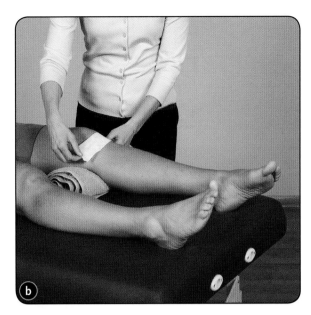

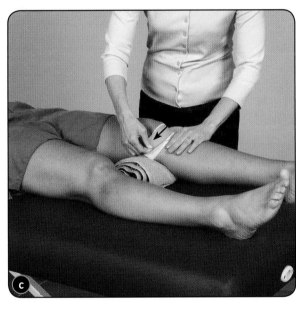

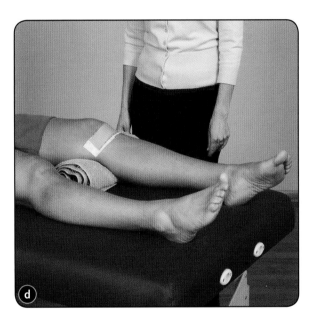

INFRAPATELLAR FAT PAD UNLOADING

Indications

This technique is effective for treating anterior knee pain, infrapatellar pain, and patellar tendinitis.

Client's Position

The client is lying or long sitting on a table, with a rolled towel or small bolster under the knee (30 degrees of flexion).

Physical Therapist's Position

The PT is standing, facing the affected leg.

Screen

Perform the infrapatellar fat pad unloading test (*a*): If pain is present in the infrapatellar area, offload the medial and lateral infrapatellar fat pads by applying a superior force under the fat pads. If symptoms decrease with the provoking activity, apply this taping technique.

Application Guidelines (McConnell)

1. Start underwrap tape at the tibial tubercle, and create a wide V to the lateral and medial joint lines (*b*).

2. Start strapping tape at the bottom of the V, following the underwrap. As the strapping tape is pulled toward the joint line, the underwrap will crease, allowing the fat pad to unload (*c*).

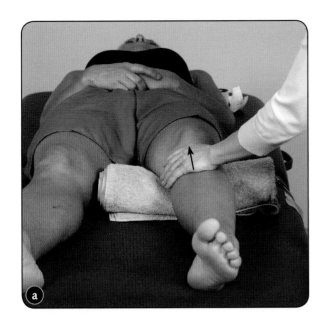

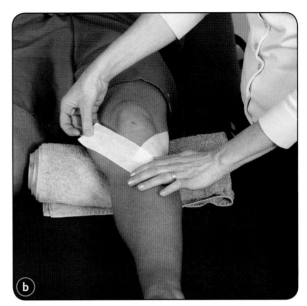

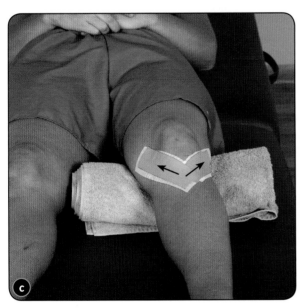

PES ANSERINUS BURSITIS
UNLOADING

Indication

This technique is effective for treating medial knee pain around the adductor bursa.

Client's Position

The client is long sitting on a table.

Physical Therapist's Position

The PT is standing, facing the affected leg.

Screen

Perform the pes anserinus unloading test (a): Offload the medial (pes anserinus) tendinous attachments by applying a compressive force superior to or inferior to the medial joint line.

Application Guidelines

1. The taping technique is similar to patellar tendon unloading, starting at the medial calf and pulling anteriorly to the midline of the shin (b).

2. An alternative technique is to place the tape just superior to the joint line and pull posteriorly, or make a V strip (as in intrapatellar fat pad unloading technique) (c).

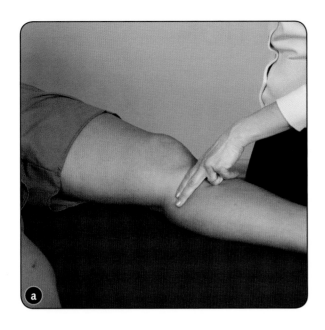

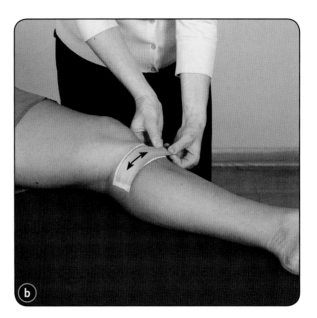

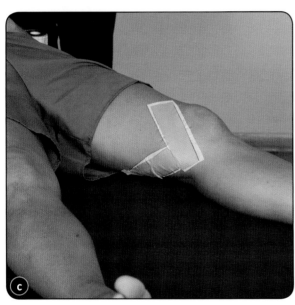

ILIOTIBIAL BAND (ITB) FRICTION SYNDROME

Indications

This technique is effective for treating lateral knee pain and ITB tightness.

Client's Position

The client is lying or long sitting on a table.

Physical Therapist's Position

The PT is standing, facing the affected leg.

Screen

Perform the ITB unloading test, similar to the pes anserinus unloading test but for the lateral knee (*a*).

Application Guidelines

1. The taping technique is similar to fat pad unloading, but the V is applied to the lateral knee above and below the lateral joint line, approximately 2 inches (5 cm) proximal on the femur and distal on the tibia (*b*).

2. An alternative technique is to use an unloading horizontal strip superior to the joint line and pulling posteriorly, similar to the pes anserinus unloading technique (*c*).

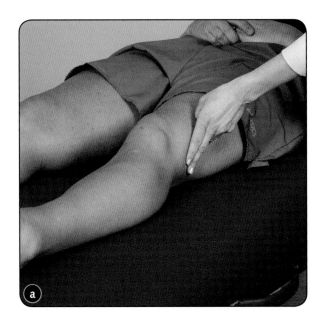

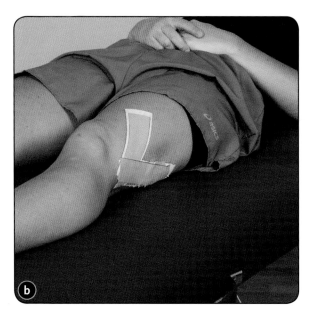

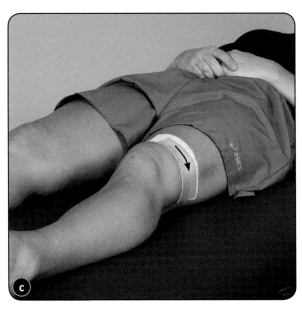

PROXIMAL FIBULAR GLIDE

Indication

This technique is effective for treating lateral knee pain.

Client's Position

The client is standing.

Physical Therapist's Position

The PT is standing, facing the affected leg. A second clinician is required to assist with taping.

Screen

For pain in the lateral knee distal to the joint line, perform the proximal fibular glide test (*a*): Apply force to the proximal fibular head, and glide anteriorly. If this decreases symptoms, apply this taping technique.

Application Guidelines (Mulligan)

1. Locate the proximal fibula, and glide the fibular head forward.
2. The second clinician starts underwrap posterior to the fibular head (*b*).
3. Apply strapping tape, pulling anteriorly around the tibial tubercle and anchoring on the medial tibia (*c-d*).

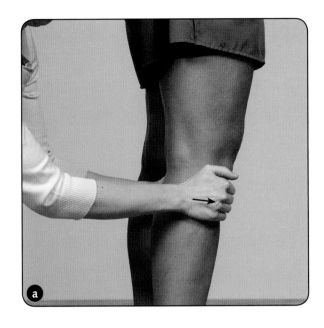

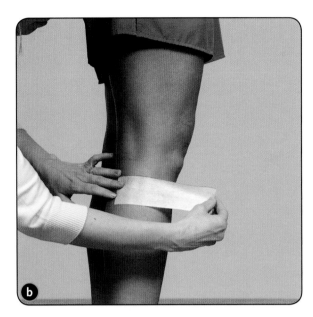

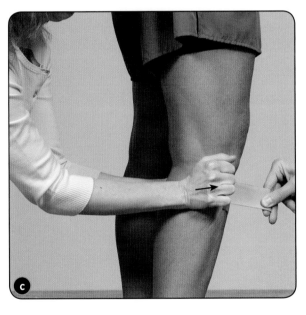

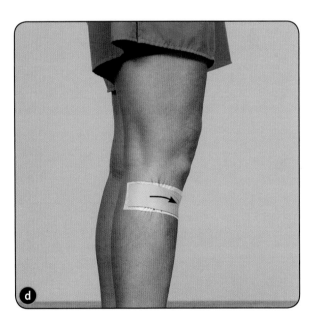

TIBIOFEMORAL TORSION

Indications

This technique is effective for treating anterior knee pain, lacking tibial internal rotation glide, and proximal tibiofibular glide.

Client's Position

The client is long sitting on a table or standing.

Physical Therapist's Position

The PT is standing, facing the affected leg.

Screen

Perform a tibial internal rotation glide (Mulligan and McConnell). For an externally rotated tibia or laterally placed patella or tibial tubercle, place the standing knee in slight flexion and internal rotation (pronate the foot), and apply an internally rotating force at the tibial plateau. For an internally rotated tibia, try placing the tibia in external rotation, and assess if symptoms decrease; apply appropriate taping technique.

Application Guidelines (Mulligan and McConnell)

1. Start underwrap posterior to the fibular head and distal to the patella (a).
2. Apply strapping tape, proceeding anteriorly across the popliteal fossa and superiorly onto the hamstrings, extending halfway up the leg (b).

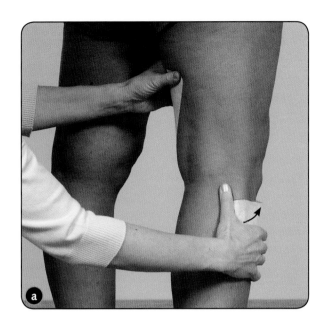 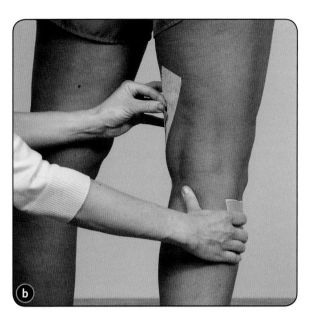

KNEE HYPEREXTENSION BLOCK

Indication

This technique limits the range of motion of knee hyperextension.

Client's Position

The client is prone with the leg extended or in slight flexion.

Physical Therapist's Position

The PT is standing, facing the affected leg.

Application Guidelines

1. Apply underwrap in the form of an X in the center of the popliteal fossa (*a*). The distance between the ends of the X and the joint line can be anywhere from 3-6 inches. The larger the X, the tighter the tape will pull to limit extension.

2. Apply strapping tape in the form of an X (*b*). Try to prevent wrinkles when applying the tape; wrinkles will cause discomfort when the patient flexes the knee.

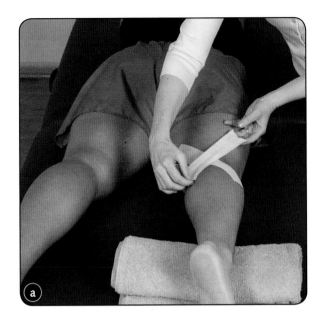 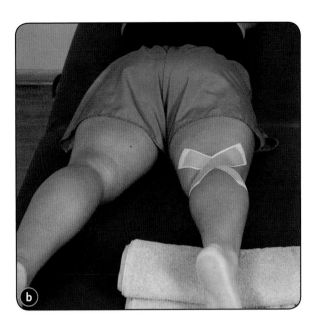

TENSOR FASCIA LATA (TFL) GLIDE

Indications

This technique is effective for treating trochanteric bursitis and lateral upper thigh pain.

Client's Position

The client is standing.

Physical Therapist's Position

The PT is standing behind the client, a second PT assists, facing the client.

Screen

Perform the TFL unloading test by offloading the TFL anteriorly and superiorly while the patient performs the aggravating activity; assess for pain relief (a).

Application Guidelines (Mulligan)

1. Anteriorly and superiorly glide the soft tissue around the greater trochanter.
2. Apply underwrap starting at the posterior superior gluteals and ending on the abdomen below the navel (b).
3. Apply strapping tape, pulling across the abdomen superiorly (c).

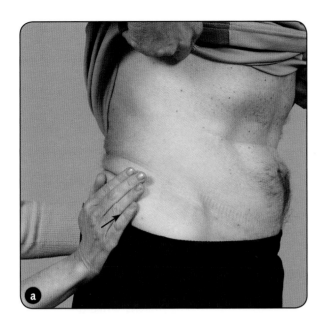

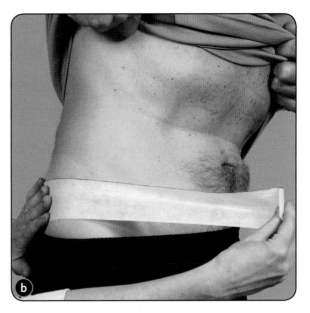

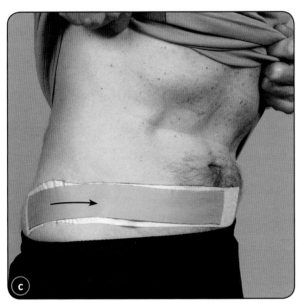

MEDIAL HAMSTRING UNLOADING

Indication

This technique is effective for treating pain in the medial hamstring during knee flexion.

Client's Position

The client is prone.

Physical Therapist's Position

The PT is standing, facing the affected leg.

Screen

Perform the medial hamstring unloading test (*a*): If pain is present in the medial hamstring with use, apply a compressive or lateral force to the muscle while the patient performs the aggravating activity. If pain decreases, this taping technique would be indicated.

Application Guidelines (Mulligan)

1. Locate the painful side, and apply force laterally on the hamstring during pain-free knee flexion.

2. Apply underwrap starting at the medial hamstring and ending on the lateral thigh (*b*).

3. Apply strapping tape to the medial hamstring, pulling the tape laterally (*c*). Anchor the tape on the lateral quadriceps (*d*).

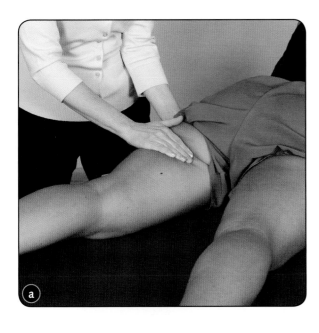

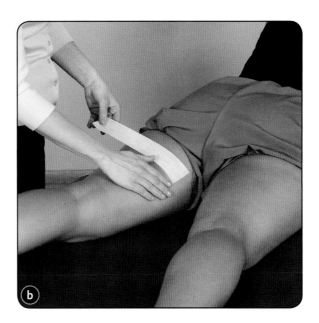

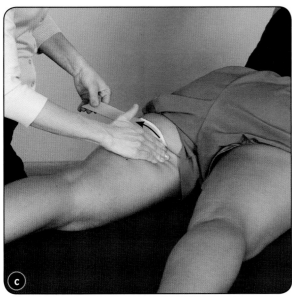

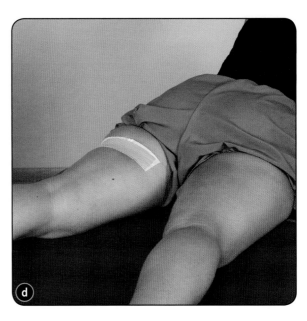

BRACES

The following braces simulate taping techniques:

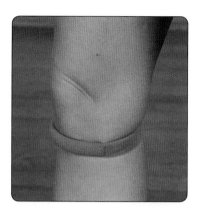

Patellar tendon strap: This off-the-shelf strap brace can be used to control pain and offload tight structures. I would rank its effectiveness for the injuries listed in the following order: patellar tendinitis, patellofemoral syndrome, infrapatellar fat pad irritation, pes anserinus tendinitis, and ITB friction syndrome.

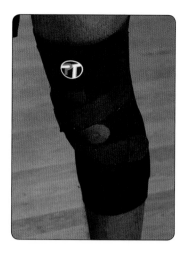

Patellofemoral syndrome braces with patellar cutout: These custom or off-the-shelf braces supposedly control patellar tracking, but I have not found them very effective because of lack of custom fit and variability of thigh sizes, especially in women.

Custom orthotics may be helpful if ankle or arch taping helps decrease knee pain.

CASE STUDIES

Taping and infrapatellar pain.

A 46-year-old female with chronic bilateral patellofemoral syndrome and X-rays showing knee and patellofemoral osteoarthritis received little relief from a physical therapy regimen of strengthening exercises and medial patellar glide taping (superior to patella). Symptoms persisted, and pain kept her from progressing in her strengthening program. She later underwent a right patellofemoral replacement. The surgery did not completely eliminate the patient's patellar pain, and symptoms were easily exacerbated by closed-chain strengthening. When the PT tried fat pad unloading taping, the patient was able to progress in quadriceps strengthening. Strength improved, and she no longer needed tape while exercising. She was able to increase strength and decrease symptoms enough to have a left patellofemoral replacement months later.

Taping and patellofemoral syndrome.

A 35-year-old male had bilateral anterior knee pain with downhill hiking only. Physical therapy included quadriceps and hamstring strengthening and core strengthening. Symptoms persisted but were reduced after strengthening. The patient received custom orthotics and reported a longer time before symptoms were experienced while hiking downhill. The bilateral knees were taped with medial patellar glide before the aggravating activity, and the patient was symptom free for an entire 6-hour hike.

The Cervical, Thoracic, and Lumbopelvic Area

The spine is a true feat of engineering—a column of vertebrae stacked on top of the sacrum to provide a balancing point for the skull, all connected by ligaments, muscles, and tendons. No wonder back pain is such a common occurrence! The areas most vulnerable to injury are typically the most mobile: the junction above the thoracic articulations with the ribs (approximately C4 to T1) and the lumbosacral junction (approximately L4 to the SI joints). The spine is truly the core of the body, and when the core is weak, it can adversely affect or cause compensations in our posture and balance as well as influence how efficiently our extremities work. Taping the spine or pelvis can be a beneficial adjunct to treatment, often correcting posture or alignment better than an off-the-shelf brace, especially if faulty posture is contributing to symptoms.

The following techniques are covered in this chapter: postural support for the cervical, thoracic, and lumbar spine; thoracic vertebra glide; rib support; low back hyperextension limit; SIJ approximation; ilial shear; diamond box unloading; and hip and gluteal muscle approximation.

Treatments are described for the following problems: SIJ pain, posture-related back and neck pain and muscle weakness, shoulder pain and impingement, instability, stenosis, spondylolysis, spondylolisthesis, low back pain related to pregnancy or obesity, rib pain and fracture, costochondritis, and sternocostal separations.

ANATOMY OF THE CERVICAL, THORACIC, AND LUMBOPELVIC AREA

The structures of the cervical, thoracic, and lumbopelvic region have a very complex interrelationship. The vertebrae of the spine articulate with adjoining vertebrae as well as the skull, ribs, sacrum, and intervertebral discs; the vertebrae also house or abut nerves, ligaments, muscles, fascia, cartilage, and arteries. The sacrum articulates with the ilia, and the ilia articulate with the heads of the femurs.

A thorough assessment of this area is needed to determine the cause of any symptoms, whether central (around the spine) or peripheral (in the extremities). Cervical, thoracic, or lumbar injuries can manifest as symptoms in the arms or legs (such as weakness, numbness, tingling, pain, or paresthesias) along corresponding nerve root distributions. Peripheral injuries can also cause symptoms of weakness, numbness, tingling, pain, and paresthesias. It is important to determine the exact location of symptom generators (and sometimes symptoms can have both central and peripheral causes).

EVIDENCE

The effect of taping on pain, especially patellofemoral pain, has been fairly well established in the literature (Conway, Malone, and Conway 1992; Bockrath et al. 1993; Cushnagan, McCarthy,

Anterior Hip and Pelvis

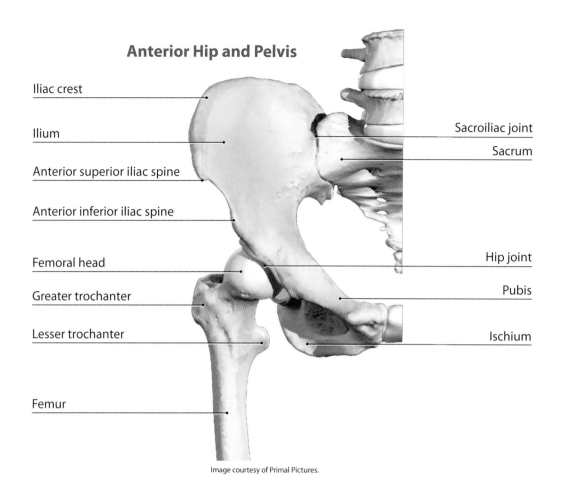

Iliac crest

Ilium

Anterior superior iliac spine

Anterior inferior iliac spine

Femoral head

Greater trochanter

Lesser trochanter

Femur

Sacroiliac joint

Sacrum

Hip joint

Pubis

Ischium

Image courtesy of Primal Pictures.

Posterior Hip and Pelvis

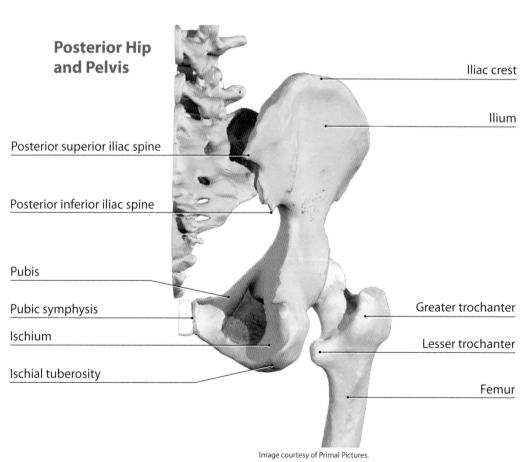

Posterior superior iliac spine

Posterior inferior iliac spine

Pubis

Pubic symphysis

Ischium

Ischial tuberosity

Iliac crest

Ilium

Greater trochanter

Lesser trochanter

Femur

Image courtesy of Primal Pictures.

Bones of the Back

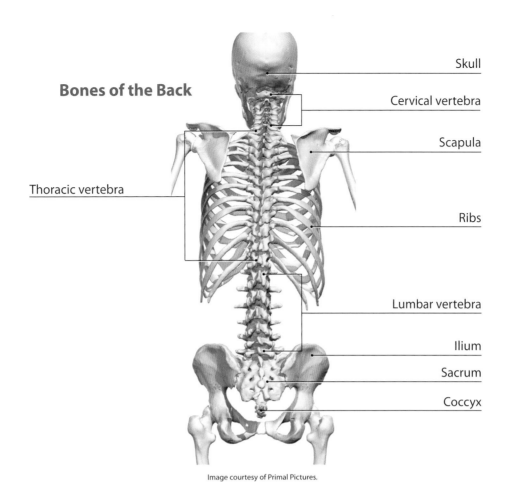

- Skull
- Cervical vertebra
- Scapula
- Thoracic vertebra
- Ribs
- Lumbar vertebra
- Ilium
- Sacrum
- Coccyx

Image courtesy of Primal Pictures.

Hip Rotator Muscles, Posterior View

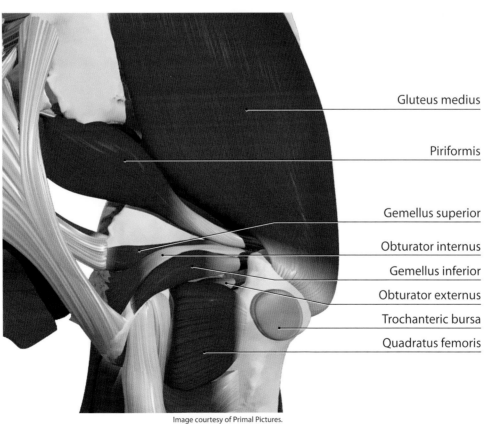

- Gluteus medius
- Piriformis
- Gemellus superior
- Obturator internus
- Gemellus inferior
- Obturator externus
- Trochanteric bursa
- Quadratus femoris

Image courtesy of Primal Pictures.

Posterior Hip Muscles, Medial View

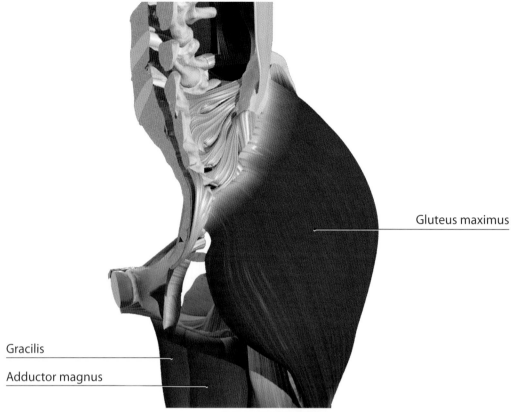

Gluteus maximus

Gracilis

Adductor magnus

Image courtesy of Primal Pictures.

Surface Anatomy, Anterior View

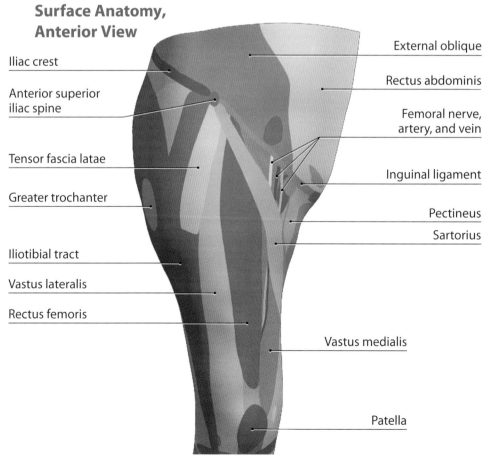

Iliac crest

Anterior superior iliac spine

Tensor fascia latae

Greater trochanter

Iliotibial tract

Vastus lateralis

Rectus femoris

External oblique

Rectus abdominis

Femoral nerve, artery, and vein

Inguinal ligament

Pectineus

Sartorius

Vastus medialis

Patella

Image courtesy of Primal Pictures.

Surface Anatomy, Back

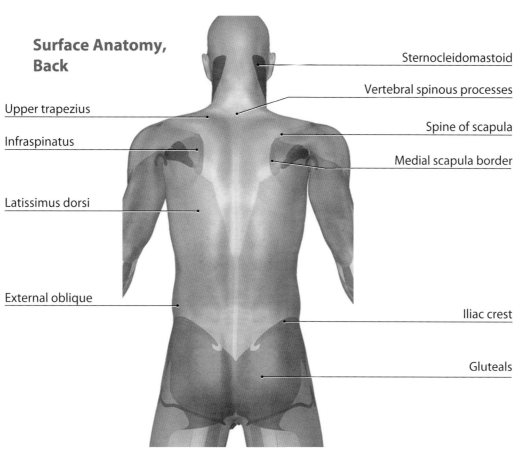

Upper trapezius

Infraspinatus

Latissimus dorsi

External oblique

Sternocleidomastoid

Vertebral spinous processes

Spine of scapula

Medial scapula border

Iliac crest

Gluteals

Image courtesy of Primal Pictures.

and Dieppe 1994; Cerny 1995; Powers et al. 1997; Gilleard, McConnell, and Parsons 1998; Cowan et al. 2002). Although there have been no studies investigating the effect of taping on low back pain, a similar pain reduction could be hypothesized. Taping the back to trigger a change of timing in the spinal musculature and thus enhance segmental stability is speculative. The unloading caused by taping enables the patient to be treated without an increase in symptoms, so treatment in general can be more effective (McConnell 2000).

Taping over the gluteus maximus is described by McConnell (2002) as a strategy to improve hip and pelvis mechanics in chronic low back pain by reducing the length of the muscle, placing it at more of a mechanical advantage. The taping may also restrict flexion, improve hip extension, or improve proprioception at the hip joint. The participants in a study by Kilbreath et al. (2006) had a history of poor chronic gait patterns. With the application of gluteal taping, participants increased their hip extension by 10°, which led to an increase in step length on the unaffected side. In another study, hip abductor taping and TheraTogs were used to increase hemiplegic hip abductor activity and gait speed during walking. Taping applied to the hemiplegic side with the hip in 5° abduction encouraged muscle facilitation (Maguire et al. 2010).

Proprioceptive taping has not been investigated with sacroiliac (SIJ) problems, but it has been reported to increase joint stability when applied to dysfunctional joints. The mechanism by which taping increases joint stability is controversial. Taping of the SIJ may aid in sacroiliac function for the same proposed reasons that patellar taping positively affects patients with patellofemoral pain syndrome (McConnell 2002).

Greig et al. (2008) describe taping as a conservative intervention that reduces thoracic kyphosis. Their study investigated the effects of therapeutic postural taping on thoracic posture in osteoporotic kyphotic women and the effects of taping on trunk muscle activity and balance; there was a significant effect, with a greater reduction in thoracic kyphosis after taping compared with both control tape and no tape. There

were no effects of taping on electromyographic (EMG) activity or balance.

In a case report by Aspegren, Hyde, and Miller (2007), a collegiate volleyball player with right anterior chest pain and midthoracic stiffness of 8 months' duration responded positively to manipulation, soft tissue mobilization, and taping.

EVALUATION

Obtain a comprehensive evaluation and history, and review any imaging studies (X-rays, MRIs, EMGs) for bony abnormalities (e.g., spondylolysis, spondylolisthesis); stenosis; and disc or nerve involvement, which may affect or direct your course of treatment. Table 4.1 provides the normal active range of motion (AROM) of the thoracic and lumbar spine and hips.

Red Flags for Taping

The following can indicate a more serious problem. It is best to refer the patient to a physician for further evaluation.

TABLE 4.1

Normal AROM of Thoracic and Lumbar Spine and Hips

Motion	Degree
Thoracic flexion	20-45°
Thoracic extension	25-45°
Thoracic side bending	20-40°
Thoracic rotation	35-50°
Costovertebral expansion	3-7.5 cm
Lumbar flexion	40-60°
Lumbar extension	20-35°
Lumbar side bending	15-20°
Lumbar rotation	3-18°
Hip flexion	100-120°
Hip extension	10-15°
Hip abduction	30-50°
Hip adduction	30°
Hip internal rotation	30-40°
Hip external rotation	40-60°

Adapted from Magee 2006

- Complaints of bowel and bladder changes
- Constant unrelenting pain or headache
- Onset of numbness, tingling, or weakness
- Increase in symptoms with cough, sneeze, or Valsalva maneuver

Strength testing should be performed to assess isometric abdominal endurance; isometric extensor endurance; and back rotator, multifidus, and hip strength as per Kendall and Kendall (1999) and Magee (2006).

Special Tests

The relevant tests applicable to evaluating the cervical, thoracic, and lumbopelvic area are:

- SIJ hypermobility testing (see Cleland 2007)
- Leg length discrepancy assessment (see chapter 3, page 56)

- Effects of manual traction (conducted on the neck or low back), which may increase or decrease symptoms
- Nerve tension testing (slump test, other upper or lower limb tension tests; see Cleland 2007)
- Cervical and lumbar instability testing (see Cleland 2007)

Biomechanical Considerations

The relevant considerations applicable to the cervical, thoracic, and lumbopelvic area are:

- Q angle of the knee (see chapter 3, page 55)
- Foot position (see chapter 2, page 17)
- Step-up and step-down mechanics (see chapter 3, page 56)
- Hypermobility joint protection and posture; common positions assumed during the day

Technique	Screening tool
Thoracic vertebra glide	Thoracic rotational mobilization with movement
Ilial shear	Ilial accessory movement

POSTURAL TAPING: UPPER BACK, MIDBACK, AND LOWER BACK

Indications

These techniques are effective for treating posture-related back and neck pain and muscle weakness, shoulder pain or impingement, and low back pain related to pregnancy or abdominal obesity.

Client's Position

The client is sitting on a table.

Physical Therapist's Position

The PT is standing behind the client.

Application Guidelines

Taping can enhance kinesthetic awareness of neutral posture, something a brace cannot do. The tape helps correct bad postural habits and promotes upper trapezius relaxation. Place the patient in an optimal neutral posture before taping: While looking at the patient from the side, imagine a plumb line from the ear to midshoulder (with the scapula retracted) to the midline of the hip, knee, and ankle.

Upper Back and Neck

1. Apply underwrap in the form of an X while the patient is sitting. Start at the upper trapezius and move toward the contralateral lower thoracic area.
2. Apply strapping tape starting at the shoulder. Pull with some force to follow the underwrap (*a*).
3. If the patient has complaints of neck pain or symptoms, another strip of underwrap starting from the center of the X can be placed up to the hairline.
4. To correct a forward head position, have the patient tuck the chin and apply a strip of strapping tape at the neck and pull down with force to meet the center of the X (*b*).

Midthoracic and Lumbar Area

1. Apply underwrap in the form of an X while the patient is sitting. Start at the mid-scapula and move toward the contralateral iliac crest or more distal depending on where the symptoms are.
2. Apply strapping tape starting at the scapula. Pull with some force to follow the underwrap (*c*).

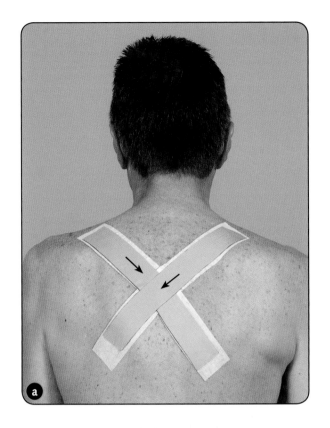

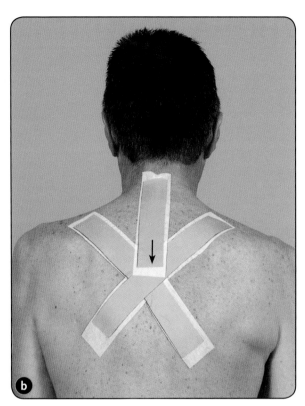

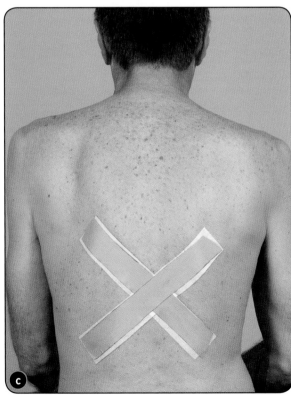

THORACIC VERTEBRA GLIDE

Indications

This technique is effective for treating thoracic and rib pain as well as pain or limitation with cervical rotation.

Client's Position

The client is sitting.

Physical Therapist's Position

The PT is standing behind the client.

Screen

Perform a thoracic vertebral correction (*a*): If accessory motion, overpressure, or mobilization with movement (MWM) of T5 and above decreases symptoms of cervical rotation restriction or pain in the upper thoracic area, apply this technique.

Application Guidelines (Mulligan 1999)

1. Ask the patient to retract the affected scapula. Apply underwrap, starting at the midline of the scapula (*b*).

2. Apply strapping tape, pulling to the direction (right or left) that improves symptoms (*c*). Anchor the tape on the other scapula (*d*).

3. Alternatively, to maintain the rotational correction, apply H strips across the mobilized area; the center of the H is on the vertebral process that is mobilized (*e*). Or apply tape in an X, with the center at the level mobilized (*f*).

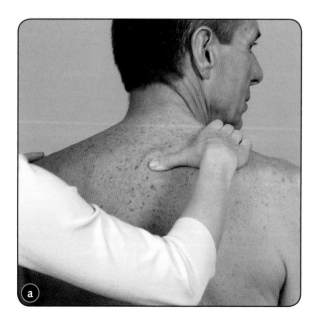

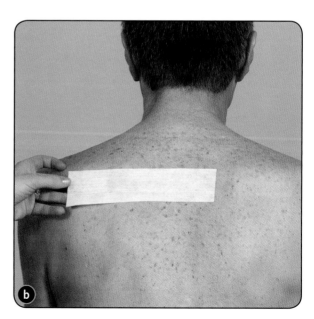

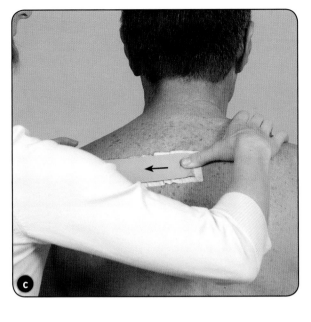

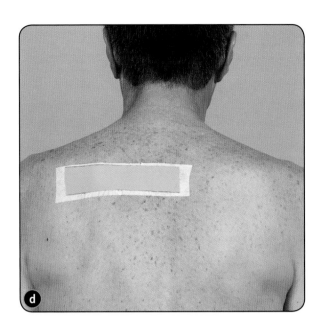

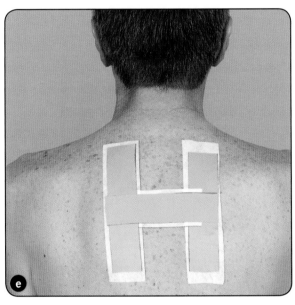

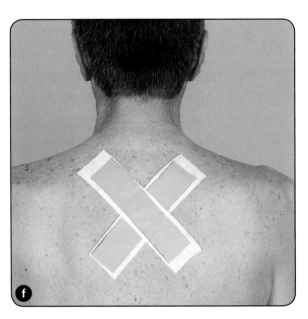

89

RIB SUPPORT

Indications

This technique is effective for treating rib pain and fractures, costochondritis, and sternocostal separations.

Client's Position

The client is prone, side lying, or supine (depending on rib area affected).

Physical Therapist's Position

The PT is standing, facing the affected side.

Application Guidelines

1. Apply underwrap in an approximately 6-inch (15 cm) strip (depending on patient's size) in an asterisk pattern around the involved rib area (*a*).

2. Apply strapping tape over the underwrap, with or without a pulling force (depending on which gives the patient most relief) toward the affected rib (*b*).

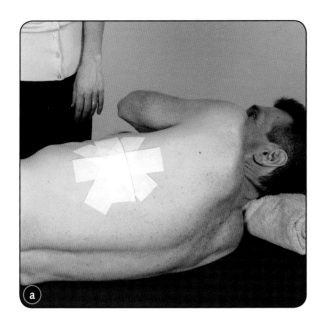 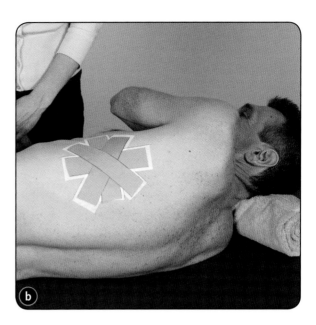

LOW BACK
HYPEREXTENSION LIMIT

Indications

This technique is effective for treating instability, stenosis, spondylolysis, spondylolisthesis, and back pain related to obesity.

Client's Position

The client is standing.

Physical Therapist's Position

The PT is standing, facing the patient's affected side.

Application Guidelines

1. Apply two parallel strips of underwrap from the anterior superior iliac spine (ASIS) level toward the lower rib angles. For further extension protection, have client stand with a posterior pelvic tilt prior to applying tape.

2. Apply strapping tape, starting caudally with desired force up to the ribs. Do not apply tape so forcefully that it limits rib excursion needed for breathing or causes the patient to assume a slouched posture in order to be comfortable.

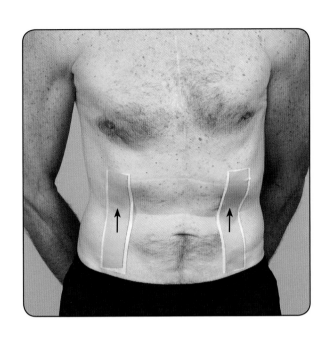

SACROILIAC JOINT (SIJ) APPROXIMATION

Indications

This technique is effective for treating low back pain, SIJ pain, and low back pain related to pregnancy or obesity.

Client's Position

The client is standing.

Physical Therapist's Position

The PT is standing behind the client.

Application Guidelines (Adapted From Mulligan and McConnell)

1. This taping technique works similar to an SI belt, relieving symptoms by physically approximating (compressing) the SI joint. Start applying underwrap at the iliac crest, moving toward the contralateral side and crossing over the sacrum to form an X (a).

2. Apply two or three strips of strapping tape with force, pulling inferiorly and laterally (b-c).

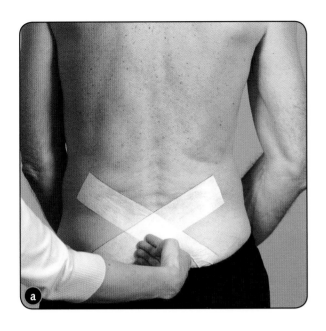

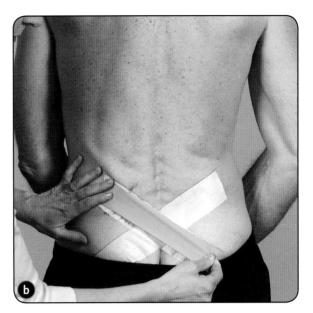

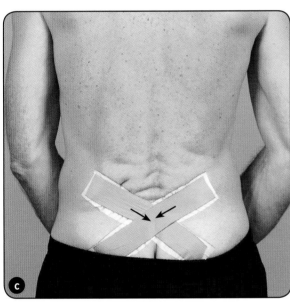

ILIAL SHEAR, ANTERIOR OR POSTERIOR

Indication

This technique is effective for treating SIJ pain.

Client's Position

The client is standing.

Physical Therapist's Position

The PT is standing or squatting next to the affected side. A second person is needed (standing) to assist with this technique to help anchor the tape.

Screen

Assess whether shearing the ilium (by providing forceful anterior or posterior glide of the ilium on the sacrum [a]) decreases symptoms, and then tape accordingly.

Application Guidelines (Mulligan)

1. If the anterior ilial position improves symptoms, enlist the help of a second clinician to anteriorly shear the patient's ilium in preparation for taping.

2. Apply underwrap, starting at the PSIS and pulling toward the contralateral ASIS ending on the abdomen (b).

3. Apply two or three strips of strapping tape, with force, while the second clinician continues to hold the patient's ilium in a anteriorly sheared position (c-d).

4. If the posterior ilial position improves symptoms, the second clinician shears the patient's ilium posteriorly.

5. Apply underwrap and strapping tape, beginning anterior to the ASIS and pulling with force toward the contralateral lumbar spine and anchor there.

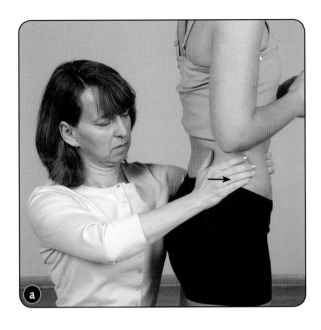

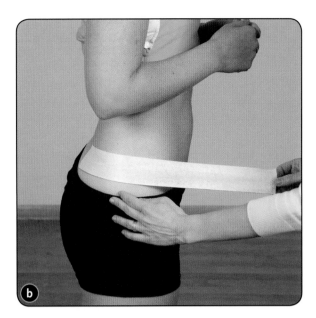

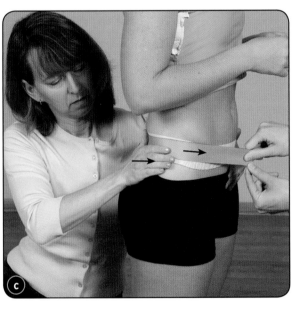

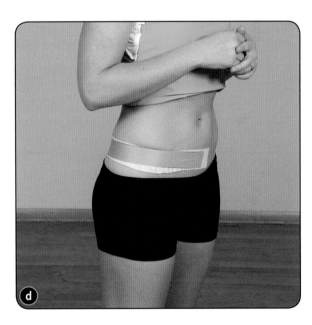

DIAMOND BOX UNLOADING

Indication

This technique is effective for treating radicular low back pain.

Client's Position

The client is standing.

Physical Therapist's Position

The PT is standing behind the client.

Screen

If approximating the soft tissues of the gluteals, hamstrings, or calf improves radicular symptoms, then this technique may be helpful.

Application Guidelines (McConnell 2000)

1. For gluteal unloading taping, first apply three pieces of underwrap while supporting the gluteals: (1) from the medial aspect of the gluteal fold, pulling laterally and superiorly toward the greater trochanter (*a*); (2) from the medial aspect of the gluteal fold to the top of the buttock above the gluteus maximus muscle belly, lifting it; and (3) from the superior end of the second piece of tape to the greater trochanter (Kilbreath et al. 2006).

2. Apply strapping tape with tension over the underwrap, three pieces as in step one (*b*).

3. For radicular unloading: Tape down the leg with underwrap and strapping tape, following the dermatome to offload the inflamed tissue.

4. Place a diagonal strip of tape midthigh over the appropriate dermatome (e.g., posterior thigh for S1; lateral aspect of the thigh for L5), lifting the soft tissues superiorly toward the buttock (*c*). The direction of the tape is dependent on symptom response. If there is an increase in symptoms, reverse the direction of the diagonal.

5. Apply another diagonal piece of tape, starting at midcalf or midshin (following the dermatome), lifting the skin superiorly (*d*). The tape is kept on for a week; usually only two or three applications are needed before the symptoms are well controlled (McConnell 2002).

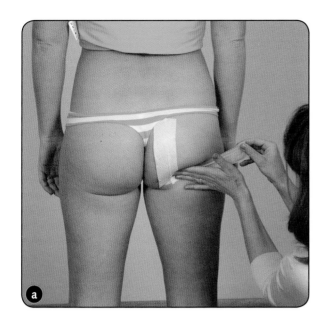

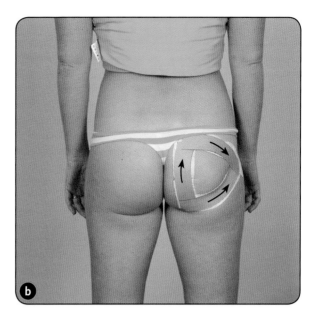

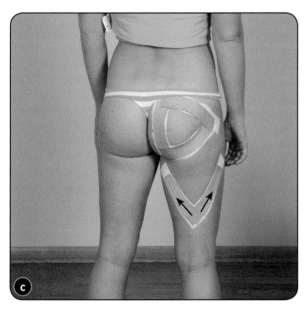

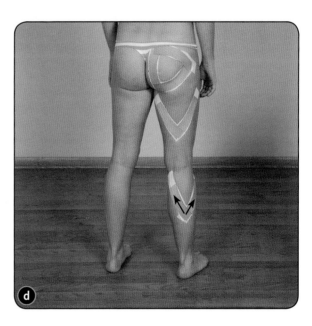

HIP AND GLUTEAL MUSCLE APPROXIMATION

Indications

This technique is effective for treating tonal changes in the lower extremity or hip musculature and gait deviation due to limited gluteal activation.

Client's Position

The client is standing.

Physical Therapist's Position

The PT is standing, facing the affected side of the client.

Application Guidelines

1. Apply three bands of underwrap, starting just below the greater trochanter and moving

   ■ directly upward to the iliac crest,

   ■ upward and anteriorly to the ASIS, and

   ■ upward and posteriorly toward the posterior third of the iliac crest (Maguire 2009) (*a*).

2. Follow with three pieces of strapping tape, using and upward pull (*b*).

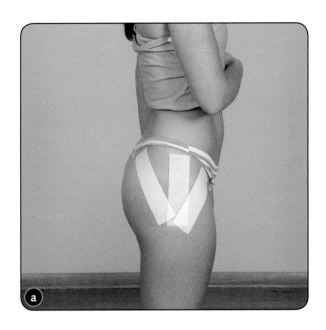 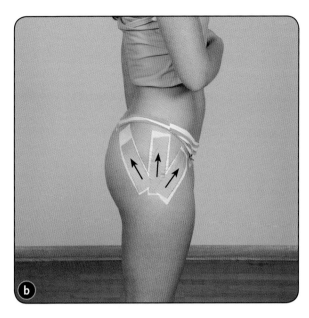

BRACES

The following braces simulate taping techniques:

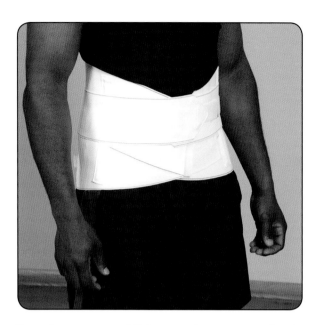

Lumbar corset: This over-the-counter elastic or semirigid brace is used to offload the back musculature or provide upright postural cues, especially with standing, bending, and lifting activities.

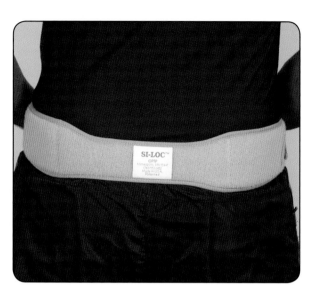

Sacroiliac belt: SI belts are worn at the level of the SI joints to provide a compression stability of the iliosacral area, mostly during standing and walking activities. They are available at medical supply stores that sell to the public.

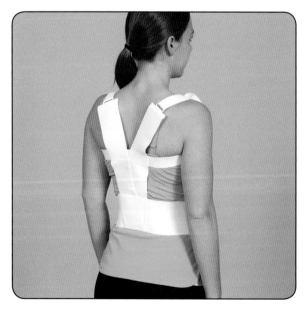

Posture brace: I have not found these to be either comfortable or effective overall because of their bulkiness and the variability of patient body types. They are available in medical supply stores and sometimes over the counter.

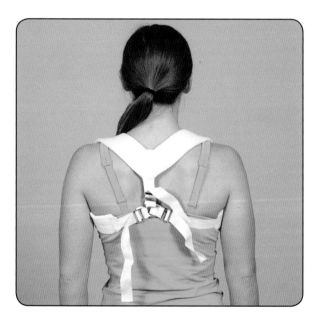

Figure eight brace: As with the posture brace, I have not found these to be either comfortable or effective overall because of their bulkiness and the variability of patient body types. They are available in medical supply stores and sometimes over the counter.

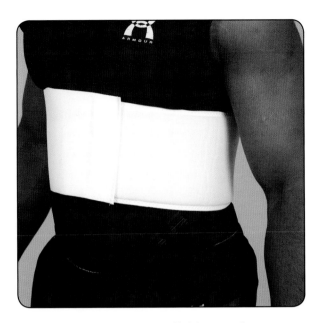

Rib belt: Rib belts are available over the counter or in medical supply stores to stabilize an injured or fractured rib.

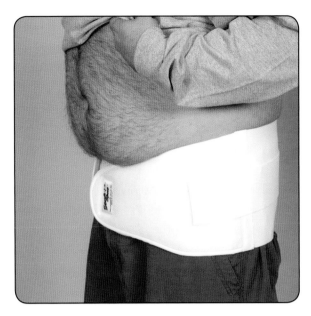

Pregnancy or obesity support belt: This elastic brace, available over the counter or in medical supply stores, is worn under the belly to help support its weight.

CASE STUDIES

Postural back taping and neck or midback pain.

A 37-year-old male had bilateral upper- and midthoracic pain, and his job requires significant time using a computer. He also had two young children he was constantly bending over to lift up, using poor body mechanics of increased thoracic flexion. He reported an immediate significant decrease in pain during the workday with postural taping and mostly muscle fatigue at the end of the workday. I recommended an ergonomic evaluation for work because he was more than 6 feet (183 cm) tall and was compensating for his small desk, which was designed for a shorter coworker. He raised the computer screen to encourage upright posture; got a headset and an adjustable keyboard tray with a mouse extension; and then worked on postural strengthening, stretching, and applied postural back taping with relief of symptoms.

Postural low back taping.

A 28-year-old female student involved in a motor vehicle accident presented with low back pain. She had a previous history of a herniated disc at L4 during birth of a child. She had severely tight hamstrings, decreased lumbar lordosis, and significant paraspinal muscle tightness and guarding. She was taped in prone from the thoracolumbar junction to the SIJ to encourage her position of relief, which was extension. She reported immediate relief while sitting in class and had improved awareness of the anterior pelvic tilt position. She continued physical therapy for lumbar stabilization, joint mobilization, and symptom control.

The Shoulder

he shoulder is another area where taping is very effective because of the relatively superficial acromioclavicular (AC) joint and the ease of correcting the poor posture (rounded shoulders and forward head) that can contribute to shoulder impingement and other shoulder problems. Postural taping is usually the first technique I apply in the clinic for clients with shoulder symptoms.

The following techniques are covered in this chapter: postural upper back (see also chapter 4), AC joint separation and clavicle fracture correction, AC joint blocking, scapula position correction, inferior subluxing shoulder correction, and anterior shoulder dislocation protection.

Treatments are described for the following problems: acromioclavicular impingement, separation, or crepitus; rotator cuff tendinitis or impingement; subacromial bursitis; anterior shoulder tightness or pain; ligamentous laxity or subluxation; cervicothoracic problems; thoracic outlet syndrome (TOS); headaches; the forward head and rounded shoulder posture that contributes to symptoms; and postural upper back weakness.

ANATOMY OF THE SHOULDER

The shoulder is a complex structure that consists of various joints (the glenohumeral joint, the acromioclavicular joint, the sternoclavicular joint, and the scapulothoracic joint), ligaments, a joint capsule, a glenoid labrum, muscles, tendons, and soft tissue structures (bursae, discs) that permit a great deal of mobility without sacrificing stability. According to Lewis, Wright, and Green (2005), subacromial impingement syndrome is one of the most common forms of shoulder pathology; pain and dysfunction occur when the shoulder is placed in positions of elevation. Rotator cuff muscle weakness and alterations in bony alignment of the shoulder girdle can also put the shoulder at risk for injury (Hertling and Kessler 1996) when normal biomechanics are altered or compensation patterns exist.

EVIDENCE

Taping and shoulder impingement. Taping is useful for addressing movement faults at the scapulothoracic, glenohumeral, and acromioclavicular joints. The exact mechanism by which shoulder taping is effective is not yet clear, but the hypothesis is that the effects are both proprioceptive and mechanical (Alexander et al. 2003). In a study by Bennell et al. (2007), of 10 physiotherapists in Australia who were considered experts in treating shoulder conditions, 50% use taping in combination with other treatment modalities for chronic rotator cuff symptoms. Another study by Miller and Osmotherly (2009) provides preliminary evidence of a short-term role for scapular (postural) taping in addition to routine physical therapy in the management of shoulder impingement symptoms.

Two studies examined using tape to provide structural support for patients with orthopedic injuries. Host (1995) applied tape every 4 days to a patient with anterior impingement syndrome to hold the scapula in proper alignment. The tape was discontinued when the patient could flex and abduct the arm and perform the home exercise program without pain. It was proposed that scapular taping be used as an adjunct therapy to attain a more favorable scapular alignment.

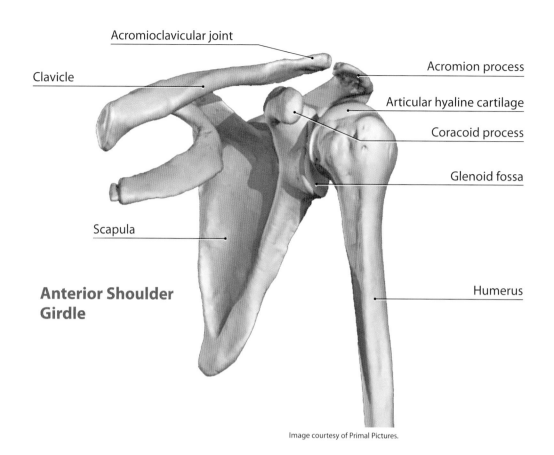

Acromioclavicular joint

Clavicle

Acromion process

Articular hyaline cartilage

Coracoid process

Glenoid fossa

Scapula

Anterior Shoulder Girdle

Humerus

Image courtesy of Primal Pictures.

Shoulder Complex Ligaments

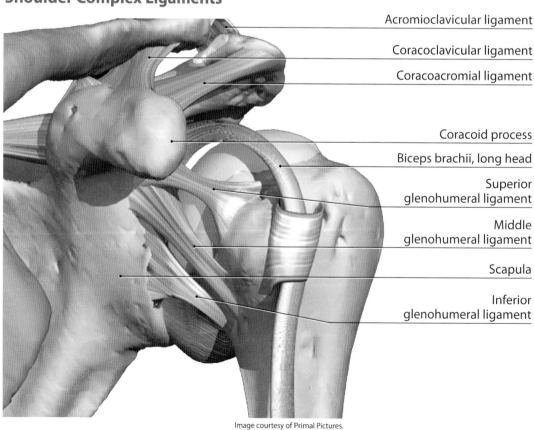

Acromioclavicular ligament

Coracoclavicular ligament

Coracoacromial ligament

Coracoid process

Biceps brachii, long head

Superior glenohumeral ligament

Middle glenohumeral ligament

Scapula

Inferior glenohumeral ligament

Image courtesy of Primal Pictures.

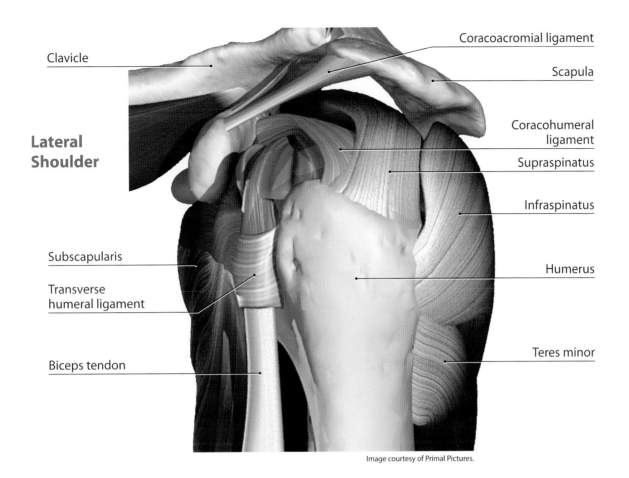

Lateral Shoulder

Clavicle

Coracoacromial ligament

Scapula

Coracohumeral ligament

Supraspinatus

Infraspinatus

Subscapularis

Transverse humeral ligament

Humerus

Biceps tendon

Teres minor

Image courtesy of Primal Pictures.

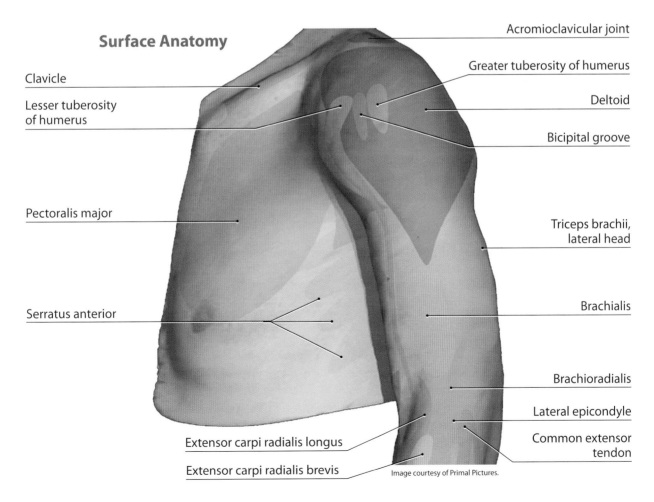

Surface Anatomy

Clavicle

Acromioclavicular joint

Greater tuberosity of humerus

Lesser tuberosity of humerus

Deltoid

Bicipital groove

Pectoralis major

Triceps brachii, lateral head

Serratus anterior

Brachialis

Brachioradialis

Lateral epicondyle

Extensor carpi radialis longus

Common extensor tendon

Extensor carpi radialis brevis

Image courtesy of Primal Pictures.

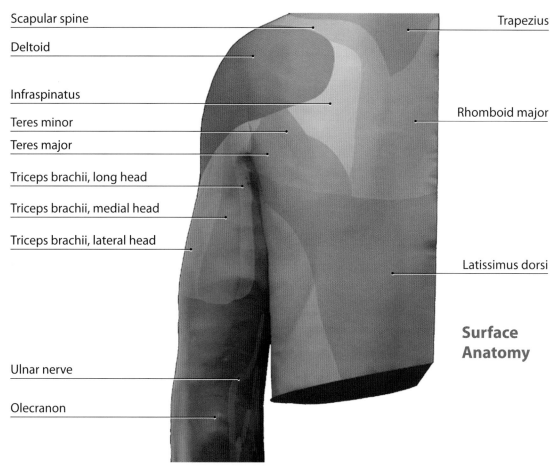

Scapular spine

Deltoid

Infraspinatus

Teres minor

Teres major

Triceps brachii, long head

Triceps brachii, medial head

Triceps brachii, lateral head

Ulnar nerve

Olecranon

Trapezius

Rhomboid major

Latissimus dorsi

Surface Anatomy

Image courtesy of Primal Pictures.

Shamus and Shamus (1997) used taping for pain management in patients with acromioclavicular joint sprains. The patients were able to discontinue use of a sling without any increase in symptoms when the AC joint was taped. Both articles illustrate the efficacy of tape to achieve improved structural support, with reported benefits of reduced pain (Peterson 2004).

Taping and posture. Changing one or more of the components of upper back and neck posture may have a positive effect on shoulder range of movement and the point at which pain is experienced, demonstrating the effectiveness of physical therapy for the management of chronic rotator cuff pain (Lewis, Wright, and Green 2005). In a study by Selkowitz et al. (2007), scapular taping decreased upper trapezius and increased lower trapezius EMG activity in patients with shoulder impingement during a functional overhead reaching task, and taping decreased upper trapezius activity during shoulder abduction in the scapular plane. In a study by Alexander et al. (2003), the application of Endura-Fix (underwrap) tape inhibited upper trapezius activity by 4%. The application of Endura-Tape (strapping tape) over the underwrap tape inhibited the trapezius on average by 22%. This inhibition did not last once the tape was removed.

Two studies showed taping was not beneficial. Taping the scapulae of violinists into a position that prevented excessive elevation and protraction while playing was not comfortable and limited playing quality (Ackermann, Adams, and Marshall 2002). A study of healthy subjects revealed no significant influence of tape application on EMG activity in the scapular muscles (Cools et al. 2002). However, scapular taping in a symptomatic sample caused a statistically significant reduction in upper trapezius activity but no change in lower trapezius or serratus anterior activity Smith et al. (2009).

Sparkes (2006) provides evidence that the McConnell scapular taping technique is appropriate for reducing upper trapezius activity in athletes with symptomatic subacromial impingement. According to Smith et al. (2009), subacromial impingement symptoms are associated with altered upper and lower trapezius muscle activity, which can be partially addressed by the application of tape. Postural tape was worn full time for 2 weeks.

Taping and other orthopedic and neurological problems. A study by Revel and Amor in 1983 showed positive results in treating TOS in combination with physiotherapy using elastic tape. Similar results were obtained by Prost in 1990 using adhesive elastic bandages to elevate the scapula in combination with other treatments for TOS (Vanti et al. 2007).

Electrical stimulation and shoulder taping in conjunction with other rehabilitation may play a role in reducing shoulder subluxation. Using strapping tape to provide structural joint support is one intervention in the management of shoulder subluxation in patients who have had a stroke. Morin and Bravo (1997) examined the use of taping and a sling to reduce shoulder subluxation in patients with hemiplegia. Taping alone was not more effective than a sling, and the combination of both was most effective, with an 86% reduction in shoulder subluxation. Three days after removing the supports, however, the improvement relative to the initial subluxation was only 1.5 mm. Ancliffe (1992) examined the effects of shoulder taping to delay the onset of pain in the shoulders of patients with hemiplegia. The subjects who were taped had a mean of 21 days before onset of pain as compared with a mean of 5.5 pain-free days for the control group.

Griffin and Bernhardt (2006) used strapping (therapeutic or placebo) for the at-risk hemiplegic shoulder and prevented or delayed development of shoulder pain better than the standard care. All strapping was maintained over 4 weeks. Patients in the therapeutic strapping group had a mean of 26.2 pain-free days, while those in the placebo group and control group had a mean of 19.1 and 15.9 pain-free days, respectively. Range of movement and func-tion improved but were not significantly different between groups.

EVALUATION

Evaluation should be comprehensive and include screening of the neck and thoracic spine. Table 5.1 provides the normal active range of motion (AROM) of the neck and shoulder.

Strength testing should be performed for the upper, middle, and lower trapezius; serratus anterior; rhomboid; and rotator cuff musculature per Magee (2006) and Kendall and Kendall (1999).

Special Tests

The following tests are useful in evaluating the shoulder.

- Impingement testing: Test to rule out labral tears (active compression test, load and shift test), impingement (Hawkins-Kennedy test, Neer test, painful arc sign), and rotator cuff tears (the empty can test) should be performed (Lewis, Wright, and Green 2005).

- Instability testing: To test glenohumeral laxity, use the apprehension test (Lo et al. 2004) and the sulcus sign (Cleland 2007).

TABLE 5.1

Normal AROM of Neck and Shoulder

Motion	Degree
Cervical flexion	80-90°
Cervical extension	70°
Cervical lateral flexion	20-45°
Cervical rotation	70-90°
Shoulder flexion	160-180°
Shoulder extension	50-60°
Shoulder abduction and scaption	170-180°
Shoulder adduction	50-75°
Shoulder horizontal adduction and abduction	130°
Shoulder external rotation	80-90°
Shoulder internal rotation	60-100°

Adapted from Magee 2006

Biomechanical Considerations

Observe the client's posture (see section on taping and posture, page 108). Assess scapulo-humeral rhythm, observing muscle sequencing from the anterior and posterior, especially with activities done frequently (such as reaching or raising the arm overhead), to ensure there is no aberrant muscle substitution patterns. Also have the client demonstrate and correct any faulty body mechanics for commonly performed activities.

Technique	Screening tool
AC joint glide	AC MWM and accessory movement
Scapular repositioning	Forward head, thoracic kyphotic posture (slouched)
Postural upper back	Poor posture

POSTURAL UPPER BACK

Indications

This technique is effective for treating cervicothoracic problems, shoulder pain, TOS, headaches, the forward head and rounded shoulder posture that contributes to symptoms, and postural upper back weakness.

Client's Position

The client is sitting on a table, maintaining good posture of the neck and upper back (neck axial extension and scapular retraction).

Physical Therapist's Position

The PT is standing behind the client.

Application Guidelines

1. Ensure the client is maintaining proper neck and shoulder retraction, avoiding a slouched posture.
2. Place two underwrap strips diagonally, starting from midway between the neck and shoulder at the upper trapezius and down to the contralateral thoracolumbar junction.
3. Reinforce with one or two strips of strapping tape, starting superiorly and pulling to create creases.
4. This should encourage neutral posture when upright.

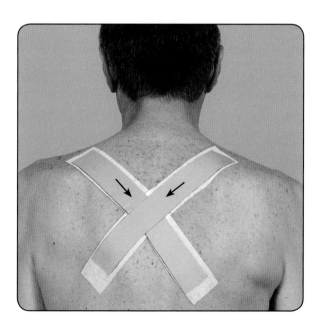

ACROMIOCLAVICULAR (AC) JOINT SEPARATION AND CLAVICLE FRACTURE CORRECTION

Indications

This technique is effective for treating AC pain or visible separation, crepitus, limited mobility of shoulder flexion and abduction above 90°, and clavicle deformity after fracture.

Client's Position

The client is sitting on a table.

Physical Therapist's Position

The PT is standing next to the affected side or sitting on the table facing the affected side.

Application Guidelines (Shamus and Shamus 1997)

1. Place a piece of underwrap the length of the inferior middle deltoid insertion to superior to the AC joint.

2. Place a second piece of underwrap from the coracoid process to the spine of the scapula (*a*).

3. Start the strapping tape at the deltoid insertion, pulling it superiorly with force to the AC joint, supporting the weight of the arm and approximating the joint (with the client's shoulder relaxed, push the humerus superiorly at the elbow). Wrinkles will appear in the underwrap if this is done correctly.

4. Place a second piece of strapping tape over the coracoid, pulling posteriorly toward the spine of the scapula, thus anchoring the first piece of tape and limiting superior movement of the distal clavicle. These two strapping pieces can be reinforced if needed (*b*).

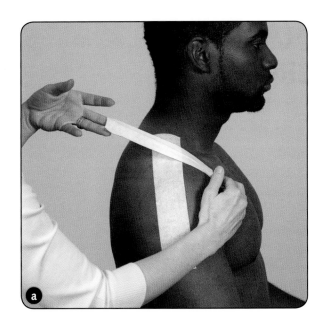 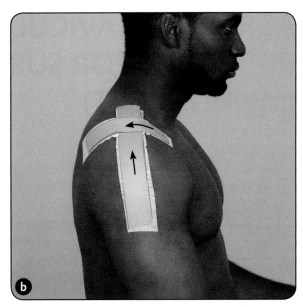

113

ACROMIOCLAVICULAR (AC) JOINT BLOCKING (FOR SUBACROMIAL IMPINGEMENT)

Indications

This technique decreases shoulder symptoms with overhead activities.

Client's Position

The client is sitting on a table.

Physical Therapist's Position

The PT is standing, facing the affected side.

Screen

Check for hypermobility in anterior or posterior glide of the AC joint (*a*), and compare with the other shoulder. If excessive or limited, then during shoulder flexion apply overpressure to the posterior glide, and see if it decreases pain (Magee 2006).

Application Guidelines (Mulligan)

1. Apply underwrap, starting at the anterior shoulder and moving toward the posterior shoulder; use approximately a 6-inch (15 cm) piece depending on the size of the shoulder and the activity (*b*).

2. Apply a second piece of underwrap, anterior to posterior medially, if needed.

3. Apply strapping tape tightly, starting at the anterior shoulder and pulling posteriorly while positioning the AC in a posterior glide (*c-d*).

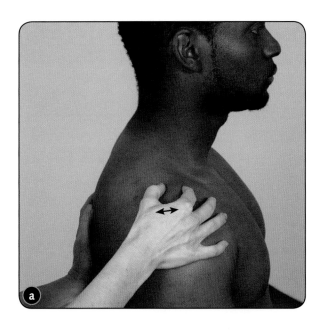

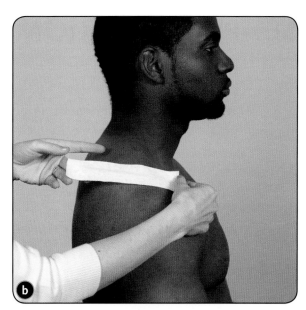

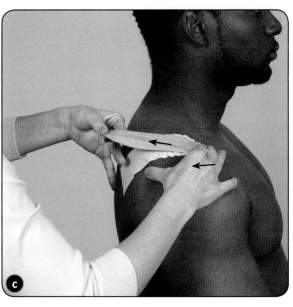

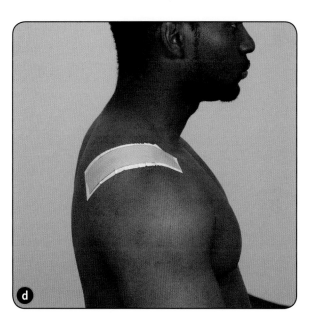

SCAPULA POSITION CORRECTION

Indications

This technique provides an alternative way to maintain neutral upper back and scapular position or to help correct poor scapulohumeral rhythm.

Client's Position

The client is standing or sitting in neutral posture.

Physical Therapist's Position

The PT is standing behind the client.

Application Guidelines (McConnell)

1. Fully retract and depress the scapula.
2. Apply underwrap from the T1 to T12 level (*a*).
3. Apply strapping tape with tension from the center of the spine of the scapula to the T12 spinous process, diagonally (*b*).

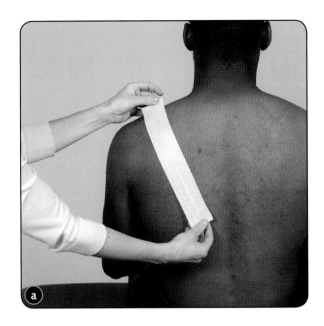 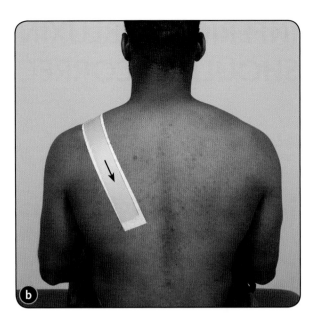

117

INFERIOR SUBLUXING
SHOULDER CORRECTION

Indications

This technique is effective for treating inferior subluxing shoulder and glenohumeral (GH) laxity (positive sulcus sign).

Client's Position

The client is sitting on a table in scapular retraction, maintaining good posture.

Physical Therapist's Position

The PT is standing next to the affected side. A second PT is needed to assist with repositioning shoulder.

Application Guidelines (Mulligan, McConnell)

1. Start with underwrap at the insertion of the middle deltoid inferiorly to proximal to the AC joint superiorly (*a*).

2. Place a second piece of underwrap from the coracoid process of the scapula anteriorly to the spine of the scapula posteriorly (*b*).

3. Start the first piece of strapping tape at the insertion of the deltoid, pulling it superiorly with force to support the weight of the arm and approximate the joint (with the client's shoulder relaxed, push the humerus superiorly at the elbow). Wrinkles will appear in the underwrap if this is done correctly (*c*).

4. Place a second piece of strapping tape over the coracoid process, pulling posteriorly to secure the tape near the spine of the scapula. This piece of tape should minimize superior translation of the distal end of the clavicle and act as an anchor for the first piece of tape (*d*).

5. Reinforce with another strip of strapping tape to extend the tape's effectiveness over time (Shamus and Shamus 1997).

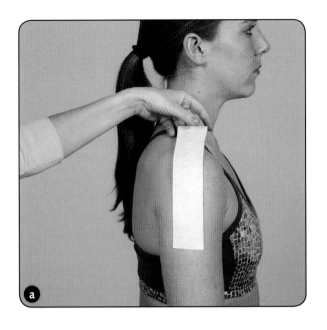

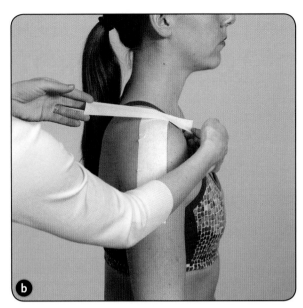

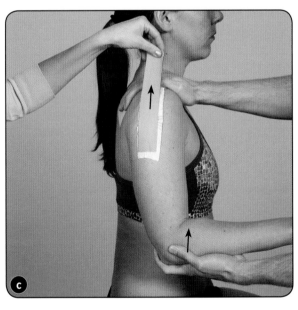

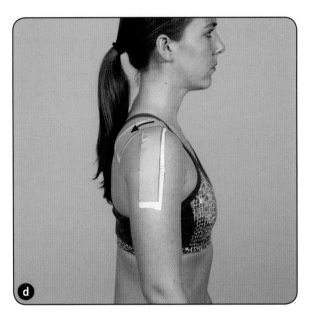

ANTERIOR SHOULDER DISLOCATION PROTECTION

Indication

This technique limits range of motion (ROM) of shoulder abduction with external rotation (anterior dislocation position).

Client's Position

The client is sitting on a table, scapula retracted, in good posture with hand on hip.

Physical Therapist's Position

The PT is sitting, facing the client's affected side.

Application Guidelines

1. Place a strip of underwrap around the upper arm (*a*), keeping the biceps tense, and a strip of underwrap from the scapula to the chest (*b*). The tape should be applied gently to prevent circulatory problems; it is used as an anchor point for the other shoulder taping techniques. Apply an underwrap piece connecting these two. Apply strapping tape over all the underwrap, using superior force with the last connecting piece (*c*).

2. Start the underwrap at the level of the biceps anchor at the posterior arm towards just distal to the AC joint, across the sternum (by following the black arrow) (*d*). Conclude this technique by firmly following the white arrow to the other anchor at the front of the chest (*e, f*). Apply another piece of underwrap at the anterior biceps anchor towards the shoulder and attach on the scapula (*f*). Make one to two crosses on the lateral deltoid to provide support, keeping the humeral head in optimal superior and posterior position. Add strapping tape to follow the underwrap (*f*).

3. Start the tape at the level of the anterior biceps anchor pulling up and over the shoulder to the posterior scapula, creating an X on the shoulder. One to three additional lines can be added for support. Each strip should partially overlap the previous strip. Add strapping tape to follow the underwrap (*g*).

4. Add straight line strips of strapping tape (no skin should be exposed at this point), beginning at the upper arm anchor, connecting to the scapular anchor by pulling superiorly in overlapping strips from the posterior deltoid (three to six strips) (*h*).

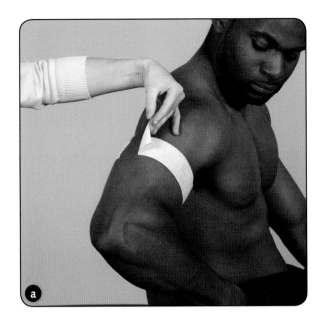

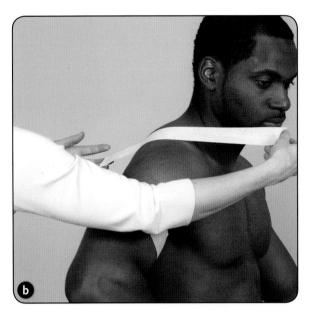

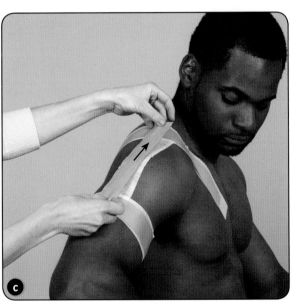

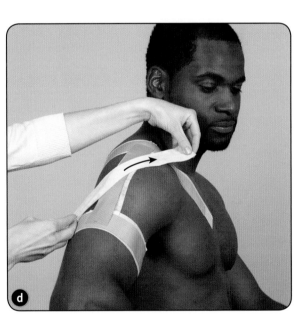

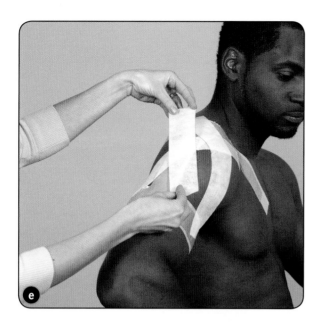

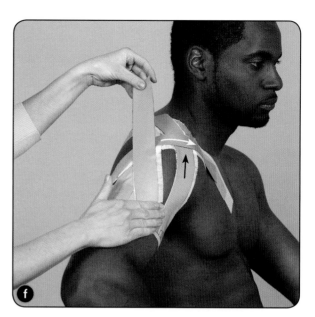

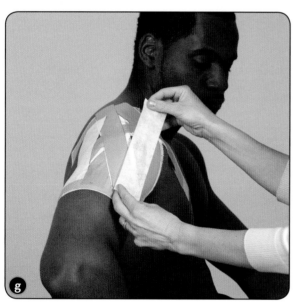

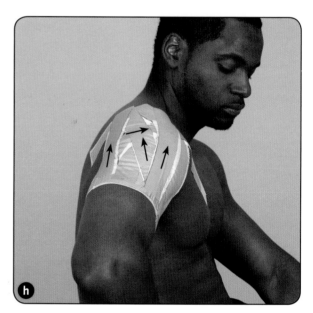

BRACES

The following braces simulate taping techniques:

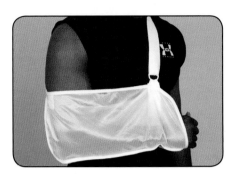

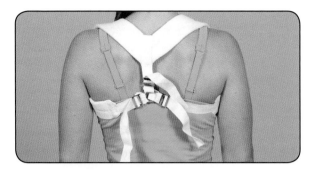

Shoulder or arm sling: Available over the counter, these slings are used primarily on the advice of a health care professional to protect against dislocation, to help support painful subluxation, or for use after shoulder surgery.

Figure eight clavicle strap or posture brace: These braces are used primarily on the advice of a health care professional after clavicle fracture or AC separation and to a lesser degree for neutral shoulder and upper back posture cueing.

AC impingement and taping.

A 37-year-old female presented after 2 to 3 months of insidious-onset left shoulder and upper trapezius (UT) pain rated 4 to 8 out of 10, worse when the hand was behind the head. She reported arm numbness, and cervical rotation and extension eased symptoms. No X-rays were taken. The patient had injured herself 6 months previously while rowing at the gym and had UT cramping; symptoms were resolved with physical therapy. She is active in weights and kickboxing and is a Pilates instructor, but she reported shoulder crepitus with these activities. Observations include slight scoliosis in sitting, unlevel pelvis, thoracic vertebral rotation, slouched forward head posture, pain with shoulder elevation greater than 150°, and normal neck movement. Resisted pain 4+ out of 5 in external rotation and shoulder abduction. Distraction of GH joint decreased symptoms with ROM. Manual cervical traction does not affect symptoms. Neck symptoms quickly resolved with ROM and elevated left first rib muscle energy correction technique. Biceps tendon irritation was 0 to 5 out of 10 after the second visit, with symptoms localized at the biceps tendon. At this point, symptoms were exacerbated only with overhead Pilates and punching. Treatment included scapular strengthening, postural taping, modified arm weight training, and iontophoresis to the biceps tendon. AC posterior glide taping resolved pain to 0 to 3 out of 10 and allowed her usual overhead activity without pain when taped only.

Taping for posture and shoulder impingement.

A 68-year-old male fell on his outstretched arm and had intermittent shoulder pain and a painful arc between 80 and 160° of elevation in flexion and abduction. Pain with resisted external rotation and abduction was present without significant weakness. He presented with slouched kyphotic posture. He was taped for posture, and immediately his painful arc decreased to 90 to 120°. He was given scapular strengthening exercises, postural correction exercises, and mobilization into posterior and inferior glenohumeral glides. Tape was used consistently for 2 weeks until he had good awareness of postural correction, especially with arm use. Upon his third visit, shoulder flexion and abduction were pain free (no painful arc was present).

The Elbow, Wrist, and Hand

The elbow, wrist, and hand can be significantly affected by taping because of the superficial nature of the joints. However, taping will limit movement of certain joints that may be necessary to carry out activities of daily living. Tape can be worn 24 hours a day, unlike many elbow, wrist, and hand splints or braces, which must be removed for bathing or doing any activity that may soil the brace (such as cooking or hobbies). The tape may need to be reapplied more frequently to the wrist and hand because it will get soiled quicker since we use our hands, especially our dominant hand, so much during the day.

The following techniques are covered in this chapter: medial or lateral epicondylitis strapping, radial head glide, diamond box unloading, ulnar ER or IR glide, elbow laxity block, neutral wrist strapping, wrist flexion or extension block, radiocarpal glide, fifth metacarpal dorsal glide, ventral ulnar glide, trapezium glide, and thumb block.

Treatments are described for the following problems: limiting elbow, wrist, and thumb ROM; medial and lateral epicondylitis; carpal tunnel syndrome; wrist sprains or pain; pronator syndrome; carpal instability; triangular fibrocartilage complex (TFCC) tears or wrist hypermobility; De Quervain's tenosynovitis; ulnar collateral ligament (UCL) tears; gamekeeper's thumb; and skier's thumb.

ANATOMY OF THE ELBOW, WRIST, AND HAND

The elbow contains the distal humerus, the proximal radius and ulna, ligaments, a joint capsule, and various muscle attachments all in close proximity to nerves. The elbow is innervated largely from C6 and C7, so it is commonly a site of referred pain from the neck. A careful evaluation and screening exam must therefore be done to rule out any neck symptom contribution to the elbow, wrist, and hand. The elbow, wrist, and hand are also susceptible to overuse or cumulative trauma injuries, which can take the form of tendinitis (medial or lateral epicondylitis) or carpal tunnel syndrome, both of which can become chronic conditions that are difficult to resolve.

The wrist joint contains the distal radius and ulna, cartilage, a meniscus, an articular disc, and eight carpal bones that along with the transverse carpal ligament create the carpal tunnel (containing arteries, flexor tendons, and the median nerve). When structures inside the narrow carpal tunnel become inflamed, symptoms of carpal tunnel syndrome can occur. The TFCC is located between the distal radioulnar and radiocarpal joints and is susceptible to injury. The distal carpal row articulates with the metacarpals, which then articulate with the bones, muscles, and ligaments of the fingers and hand.

Anterior Elbow

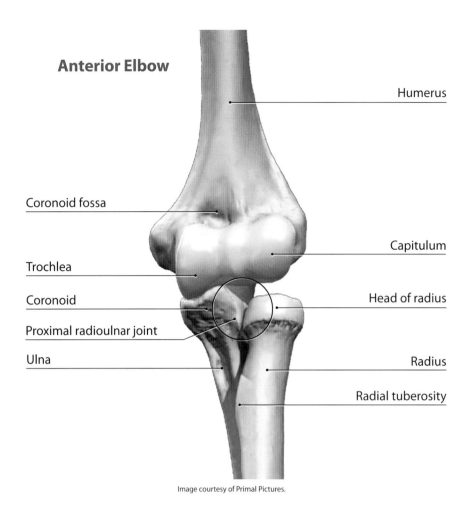

Humerus

Coronoid fossa

Capitulum

Trochlea

Coronoid

Head of radius

Proximal radioulnar joint

Ulna

Radius

Radial tuberosity

Image courtesy of Primal Pictures.

Posterior Elbow

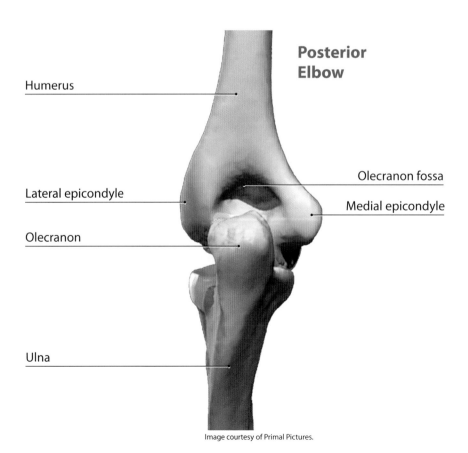

Humerus

Olecranon fossa

Lateral epicondyle

Medial epicondyle

Olecranon

Ulna

Image courtesy of Primal Pictures.

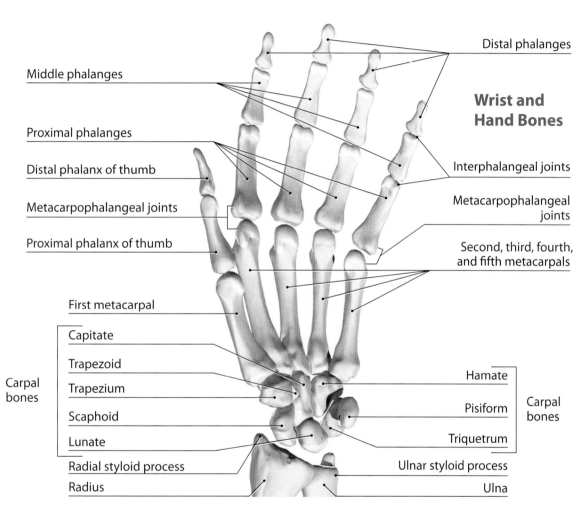

Middle phalanges

Proximal phalanges

Distal phalanx of thumb

Metacarpophalangeal joints

Proximal phalanx of thumb

First metacarpal

Carpal bones

Capitate

Trapezoid

Trapezium

Scaphoid

Lunate

Radial styloid process

Radius

Distal phalanges

Wrist and Hand Bones

Interphalangeal joints

Metacarpophalangeal joints

Second, third, fourth, and fifth metacarpals

Hamate

Pisiform

Triquetrum

Ulnar styloid process

Ulna

Carpal bones

Image courtesy of Primal Pictures.

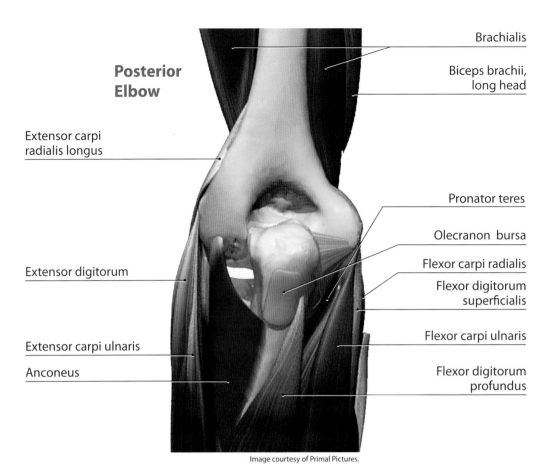

Posterior Elbow

Brachialis

Biceps brachii, long head

Extensor carpi radialis longus

Pronator teres

Olecranon bursa

Flexor carpi radialis

Extensor digitorum

Flexor digitorum superficialis

Flexor carpi ulnaris

Extensor carpi ulnaris

Anconeus

Flexor digitorum profundus

Image courtesy of Primal Pictures.

Anterior Forearm

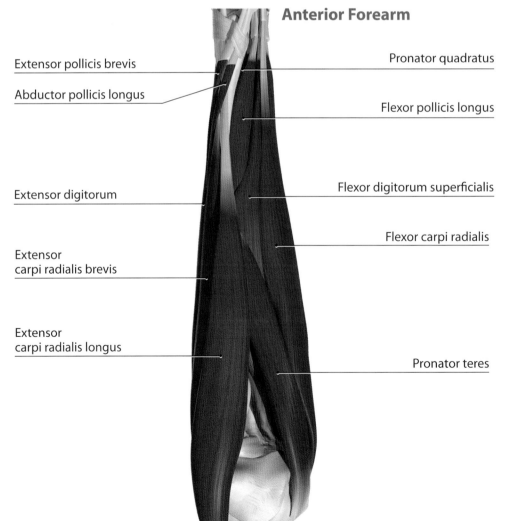

Extensor pollicis brevis

Abductor pollicis longus

Pronator quadratus

Flexor pollicis longus

Extensor digitorum

Flexor digitorum superficialis

Extensor carpi radialis brevis

Flexor carpi radialis

Extensor carpi radialis longus

Pronator teres

Image courtesy of Primal Pictures.

Posterior Forearm

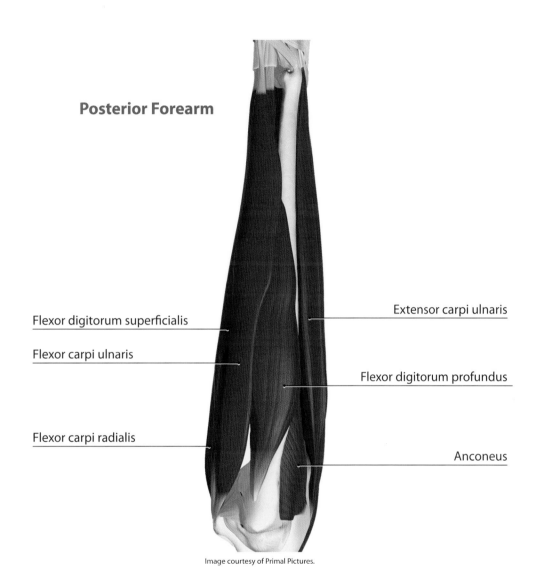

Flexor digitorum superficialis

Flexor carpi ulnaris

Flexor carpi radialis

Extensor carpi ulnaris

Flexor digitorum profundus

Anconeus

Image courtesy of Primal Pictures.

Anatomical Snuffbox

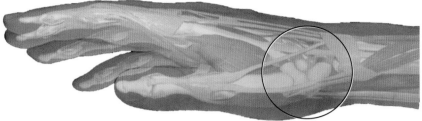

Image courtesy of Primal Pictures.

Surface Anatomy

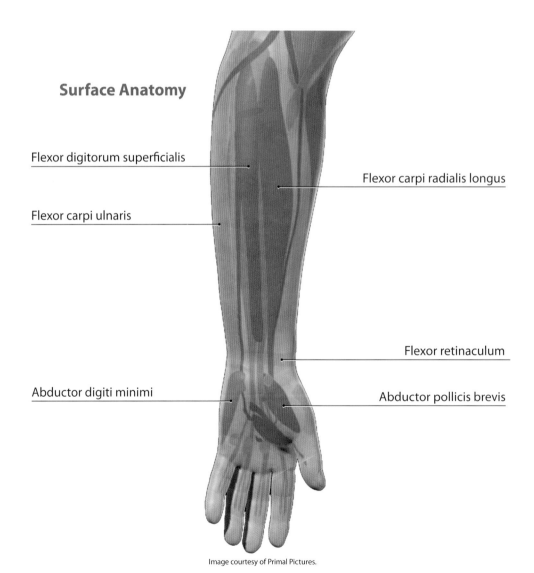

Flexor digitorum superficialis

Flexor carpi ulnaris

Abductor digiti minimi

Flexor carpi radialis longus

Flexor retinaculum

Abductor pollicis brevis

Image courtesy of Primal Pictures.

EVIDENCE

Evidence to support taping is limited in this anatomical area, but studies examining taping conducted specific to the elbow and distal were favorable. According to Vicenzino (2003), adjunct treatments such as manipulative therapy and taping techniques provide substantial initial pain relief in symptoms of lateral epicondylalgia. Early relief of pain helps accelerate recovery and motivates the client to be compliant with the treatment program. Vicenzino et al. (2003) also studied taping as related to grip strength and pain in people with lateral epicondylalgia. The taping technique improved pain-free grip strength by 24% from baseline. The treatment effect was greater than that for a placebo or control conditions. Changes in the pressure pain threshold (19%), although positive, were not statistically significant.

Schoffl et al. (2007) used a new H-taping method for flexor tendon pulley ruptures in rock climbers. The new taping method decreased the tendon–bone distance in the injured finger by 16%, whereas the other taping methods did not. Strength development was significantly better with the new taping method for the crimp grip (or hook fist) position.

EVALUATION

Before taping, it is important to assess for pain relief, accessory joint mobility, nerve compression, and instability. Screening for problems in the neck and shoulder that can refer symptoms to the wrist and hand is essential, as well as reviewing the results of any X-rays, EMGs, NCSs, and so on. Table 6.1 provides the normal active range of motion (AROM) of the elbow, wrist, and hand.

Special Tests

Extra detail is given in these tests because most physical therapists don't work a lot with hands. This material covering tests for ruling out nerve compression and tests for instability is provided as a refresher.

- Before taping the thumb: Superficial radial nerve entrapment can occur insidiously. A positive Tinel's test at the anatomical snuffbox (space between the tendons of the extensor pollicis brevis and abductor pollicis longus on the radial side and the extensor pollicis longus on the ulnar side) (Hertling and Kessler 1996) can assist with diagnosis. If radial nerve entrapment is present, ensure tape is not applied too tightly in the area of the anatomical snuffbox.

- Before taping the elbow and forearm: Perform an assessment to ensure there are no symptoms of entrapment of the radial nerve or its branches about the lateral epicondyle (Eckstrom and Holden 2002; Borkholder, Hill, and Fess 2004) because radial tunnel syndrome symptoms can mimic those of lateral epicondylitis: pain at the lateral elbow extensor mass or distal humerus, night pain, and possible paresthesias. Some potential differentiators with radial tunnel syndrome include tenderness at the neck of the radius and not the lateral epicondyle, and pain with resisted extension of the middle finger (Magee 2006).

There are three areas in the forearm that can potentially be subjected to compression. The posterior interosseus nerve can be compressed by the supinator in the canal of Frohse (a fibrous arch occurring in 30% of the population), which can lead to wrist extensor weakness. The second area of entrapment of the posterior interosseus nerve is anterior to the head of the radius by the extensor carpi radialis brevis and supinator, otherwise known as radial tunnel syndrome, which can mimic tennis elbow (Plancher,

TABLE 6.1

Normal AROM of Elbow, Wrist, and Hand

Motion	Degree
Elbow flexion	140-150°
Elbow extension	0-10°
Wrist flexion	80-90°
Wrist extension	70-90°
Forearm pronation and supination	85-90°
Wrist radial deviation	15°
Wrist ulnar deviation	30-45°

Adapted from Magee 2006

Peterson, and Steichen 1996). The last area of compression is of the superficial radial nerve by the brachioradialis, called Wartenberg's disease (Pecina, Krmpotic-Nemanic, and Markiewitz 2009); this condition is characterized by night pain at the dorsum of the wrist, thumb, and web space caused by swelling, trauma, or repetitive wrist extension activities (Magee 2006; Pecina, Krmpotic-Nemanic, and Markiewitz 2009).

With circumferential taping about the forearm, which is also performed to assist with medial epicondylitis, ensure that additional symptoms of median or ulnar nerve compression are not present under the area being taped. The median nerve can be compressed at the bicipital aponeurosis; at the proximal edge of the flexor digitorum superficialis (FDS) arch; and by the ligament of Struthers (found in 1% of the population), also called humerus supracondylar process syndrome, which can begin with sensory changes and pain and can progress to weakness. Another area the median nerve can be compressed is at the pronator teres, also called pronator syndrome, characterized by pain at the anterior proximal forearm, especially with activity. Median nerve entrapment can be tested in four ways: (1) Resist pronation with elbow and wrist flexion for 30 to 60 seconds, (2) resist elbow flexion and supination, (3) resist long finger flexion at the proximal interphalangeal joint, and (4) direct pressure over the proximal pronator teres during pronation (Butlers and Singer 1994; Magee 2006). The anterior interosseus branch of the median nerve can be compressed by the pronator as well, called anterior interosseus nerve syndrome, which is characterized by nonspecific pain in the anterior forearm, weakness in the flexors of the index finger and thumb, and inability to pinch together the tips of the thumb and forefinger (OK sign).

The ulnar nerve can be compressed at the arcade of Struthers, at the arcuate ligament, at the medial intramuscular septum, and under the fascial FDS origin, characterized by pain at the medial elbow and forearm and possible sensory deficits of the ulnar forearm into the ring and fifth finger. There can also be compression in the cubital tunnel by the flexor carpi ulnaris (FCU). This typically causes symptoms of pain or sensory changes at the medial elbow, mostly when the elbow is flexed (Magee 2006).

● Thumb ulnar collateral ligament (UCL) instability test: Apply a valgus stress to the extended thumb. A positive test shows lateral movement greater than 30°, and a partial tear is defined as greater than a 30° difference as compared with the unaffected thumb (Magee 2006).

Biomechanical Considerations

Overuse injuries to the hand, wrist, and elbow can be caused by very common activities requiring repetitive movements, forceful repeated movements, or movements routinely performed in an awkward (nonneutral) posture. It is essential to talk to patients about the activities they regularly perform and ideally evaluate them in these environments. A patient who regularly uses a computer or mouse should have his workplace evaluated ergonomically and be instructed in how to correct any discrepancies in nonneutral postures. Minor modifications to the workstation can often alleviate many symptoms (figure 6.1).

For an athlete, evaluating to ensure proper biomechanical form for the sport (e.g., whether the athlete has tennis elbow, or lateral epicondylitis) can be very helpful. Sometimes the size of the grip of an object (racket handle too large or too small) can also contribute to symptoms.

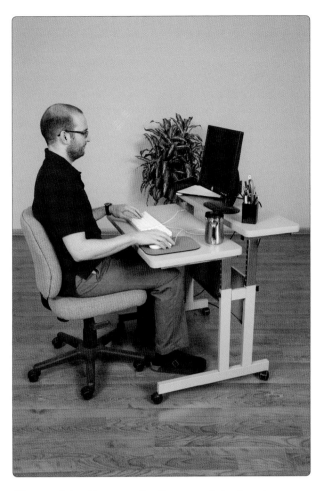

Figure 6.1 Ergonomically correct desk setup.

Technique	Screening tool

Medial or lateral epicondylitis strapping	Extensor or flexor wad unloading pain relief
	    Rule out radial nerve entrapment at proximal forearm
	    Rule out median nerve entrapment at proximal forearm
	    Rule out ulnar nerve entrapment at proximal forearm

Radial head glide	Radial head accessory movement Rule out radial nerve entrapment
Ulnar ER or IR glide	Ulnar ER or IR accessory movement
Radiocarpal glide	Radiocarpal joint accessory movement
Fifth metacarpal glide	Fourth or fifth metacarpal accessory movement
Ventral ulnar glide	Ulnar accessory movement
Trapezium glide	Trapezium accessory movement
Thumb block	UCL instability test Rule out superficial radial nerve entrapment

EPICONDYLITIS STRAPPING

Indications

This technique is effective for lateral or medial epicondylitis (pain at the medial elbow especially with flexion and pronation) and lateral or medial elbow pain with gripping activities.

Client's Position

The client is sitting with the arm on a table or is supine with the arm at the side, elbow extended.

Physical Therapist's Position

The PT is sitting at the table, opposite the client; if the client is supine, the PT is seated next to the affected arm, facing the client.

Screen

Rule out any nerve entrapment syndromes about the elbow. Perform a muscle unloading test for lateral epicondylitis (*a*): Have the patient grip forcefully. If epicondylitis is present, forceful gripping will most likely increase pain in the lateral or medial elbow (Vicenzino 2003). Apply pressure distal to the lateral epicondyle on the extensor muscles, and have the patient grip again; if pain at the elbow decreases, taping may be effective. In the presence of radial tunnel involvement, place the tape more distal on the forearm to avoid pressure on the potential anatomical compression sites. This pressure offload technique also works similarly to assess for medial epicondylitis by applying pressure to the wrist flexor group distal to the medial epicondyle while the patient exerts a forceful grip.

Application Guidelines

1. Apply underwrap approximately 1-2 inches (2.5-5 cm) distal to the elbow around the circumference of the forearm (*b*).

2. Apply strapping tape with some force (medially in this example) so that when the patient grips, the pain is decreased at the elbow and felt as tightness under the tape (*c-d*).

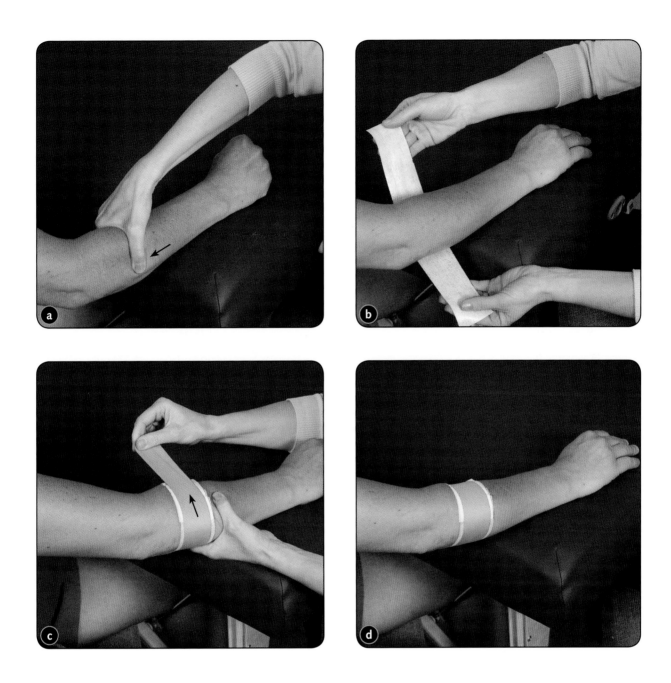

RADIAL HEAD GLIDE

Indication

This technique decreases lateral elbow pain with wrist extension.

Client's Position

The client is sitting with the arm on a table or is supine with the arm at the side, elbow extended.

Physical Therapist's Position

The PT is sitting at the table, opposite the client; if the client is supine, the PT is seated next to the affected arm, facing the client. A second clinician is required to assist with taping.

Screen

Perform the radial head accessory movement test (a) (Mulligan 1999). Biomechanically, the radial head must roll and twist with combined motions of the wrist involving flexion, extension, supination, and pronation. Sometimes the radial head gets stuck in its glide, which can contribute to pain at the lateral elbow. Have the patient perform pronation with the elbow extended; apply overpressure to the radial head medially. If this decreases elbow symptoms when gripping, a medial glide on the radius using tape could relieve symptoms. Alternatively, a sustained posterior–anterior glide overpressure on the radial head applied while the patient grips can also decrease symptoms, and tape can reinforce that position as well (Vicenzino 2003). Rule out nerve entrapment about the elbow.

Application Guidelines (Mulligan)

1. Apply the radial head glide technique before putting on underwrap.
2. Start the underwrap 1 inch (2.5 cm) distal to the elbow crease lateral to the radius (b).
3. When applying strapping tape, hold the radius in medial glide if this helps decrease symptoms (c). Pull toward the olecranon of the ulna, but do not wrap completely around the forearm.
4. If a lateral glide of the radius improves symptoms, maintain a lateral glide and then apply tape (d).

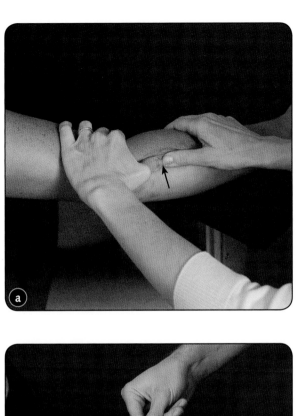

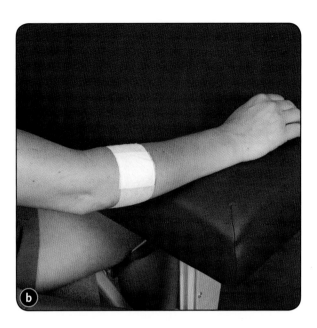

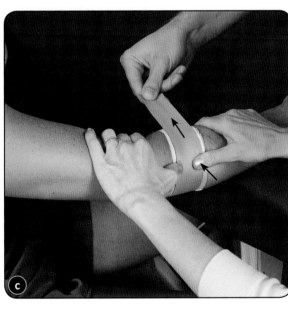

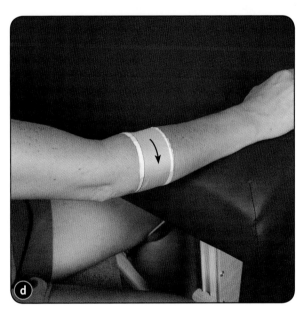

LATERAL EPICONDYLITIS UNLOADING (DIAMOND BOX)

Indications

This technique is effective for resting or night pain control of lateral epicondylitis.

Client's Position

The client is sitting with the arm on a table or is supine with the arm at the side, slightly flexed; this technique will limit some end-range motion.

Physical Therapist's Position

The PT is sitting at the table, opposite the client; if the client is supine, the PT is seated next to the affected arm, facing the client.

Application Guidelines (McConnell 2000)

1. The center of the diamond is located over the painful region. Apply the underwrap distally, anchoring it close to the midline of the forearm; it will cross the forearm diagonally (*a*).

2. Lay the underwrap down in a cephalad direction along the long axis of the arm.

3. Apply a tension force longitudinally along the direction of the underwrap so the underlying skin is approximated toward the painful region (in this case, the lateral epicondyle; *b*).

4. Reinforce with strapping tape to create a diamond shaped box around the painful area (*c*). There should be an orange peel effect present, with puckering of the skin inside the diamond (*d*).

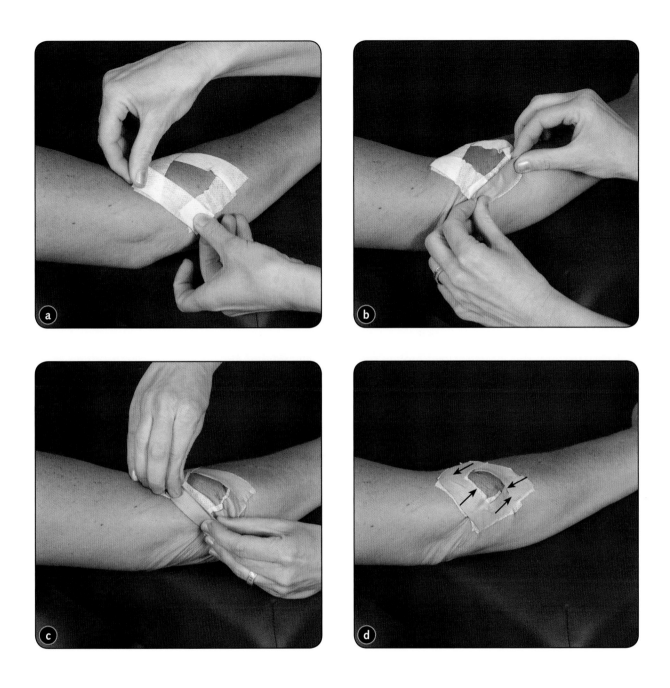

ULNAR EXTERNAL ROTATION GLIDE

Indications

This technique is effective for treating pain at the elbow or difficulty with full elbow extension.

Client's Position

The client is standing with the shoulder flexed or sitting with arm on table.

Physical Therapist's Position

The PT is standing facing the client and providing glide on the ulna and stability to the humerus. A second clinician is necessary to assist with tape pull.

Screen

Perform the accessory joint motion test, externally rotating the ulna during elbow extension (a) (Mulligan 1999). If symptoms decrease or ROM improves with external rotation (ER), this technique may be beneficial.

Application Guidelines (Mulligan)

1. For external rotation glide, apply underwrap 1 inch (2.5 cm) medial to the ulna, distal to the olecranon of the lateral forearm (b).

2. Stabilize the distal humerus with one hand while applying external rotation glide to the ulna. The second clinician pulls underwrap then half-width strapping tape under the forearm medially and then over the biceps to anchor on the lateral humerus (c).

3. Apply the second strip with more force, maintaining joint glide (d).

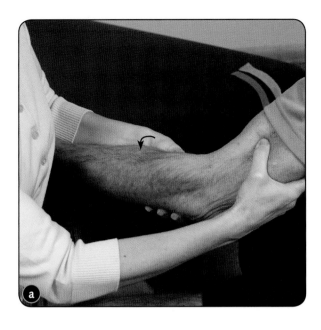

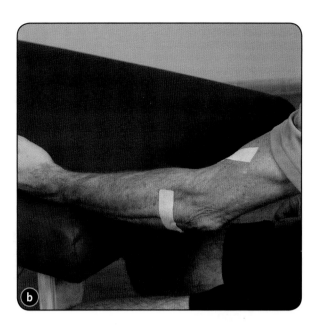

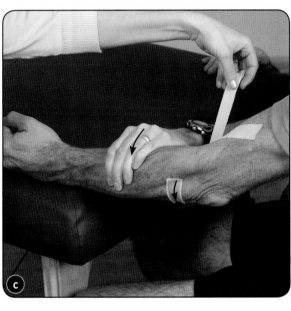

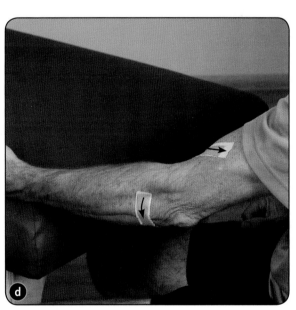

ULNAR INTERNAL ROTATION GLIDE

Indications

This technique is effective for treating pain at the elbow or difficulty with full elbow extension.

Client's Position

The client is standing with the shoulder flexed.

Physical Therapist's Position

The PT is standing facing the client and providing glide on the ulna and stability to the humerus. A second clinician is necessary to assist with tape pull.

Screen

Perform the accessory joint motion test, internally rotating the ulna during elbow extension (a) (Mulligan 1999). If symptoms decrease or ROM improves with internal rotation (IR), this technique may be beneficial.

Application Guidelines (Mulligan)

1. For internal rotation glide, maintain the joint glide and start the underwrap (b) then strapping tape 1 inch (2.5 cm) medial on the ulnar side of the forearm, with the second clinician pulling under the forearm laterally and then medially over the biceps to anchor on the lateral upper arm (c-d).

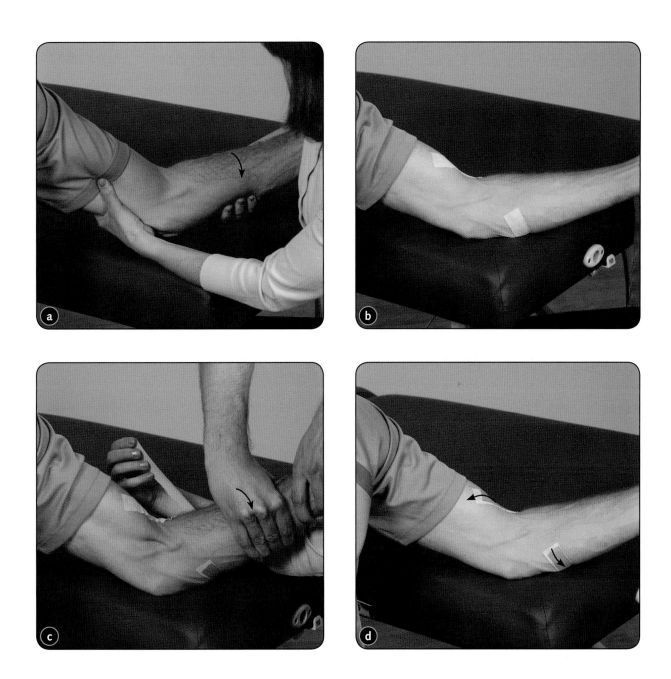

ELBOW HYPEREXTENSION BLOCK

Indications

This technique limits end-range extension or varus or valgus laxity at the elbow.

Client's Position

The client is supine. A towel may be placed under the hand to limit extension for extension block.

Physical Therapist's Position

The PT is facing the client on the affected side.

Application Guidelines

1. Apply underwrap in an X, with the center of the X on the volar elbow (for hyperextension block), medial elbow (for valgus laxity), or lateral elbow (for varus laxity) (*a*).

2. Apply strapping tape in a neutral, non-end-range position over the underwrap to limit the unwanted elbow movement (extension, valgus, or varus) (*b*).

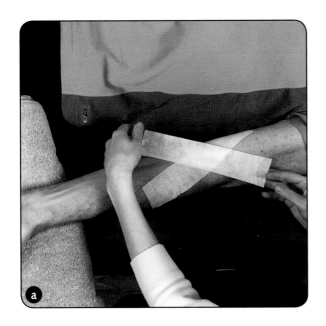

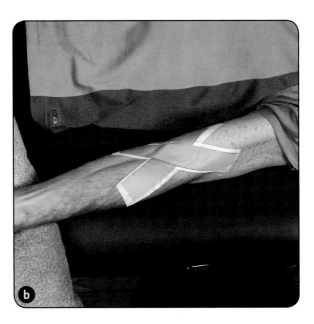

145

145

NEUTRAL WRIST STRAPPING

Indications

This technique is effective for treating medial and lateral epicondylitis, carpal tunnel syndrome, wrist sprains, pronator syndrome, carpal instability, TFCC tears, and wrist hypermobility.

Client's Position

The client is sitting with the arm on a table.

Physical Therapist's Position

The PT is sitting at the table, opposite the client.

Application Guidelines

1. Apply underwrap with the wrist in a neutral position, one strip from the dorsal midforearm to 1 inch (2.5 cm) distal to the radial styloid process, and another strip from the volar midforearm to 1 inch distal to the radial styloid process on the palmar hand. Apply a third strip around the carpals, making sure the underwrap does not compress the wrist to create or worsen hand paresthesias, pain, or other symptoms.

2. Follow with strapping tape, pulling distally (*a-b*).

3. Anchor with a strip around the wrist (*c*).

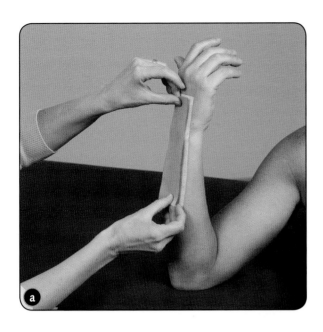

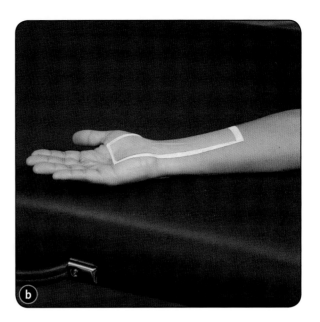

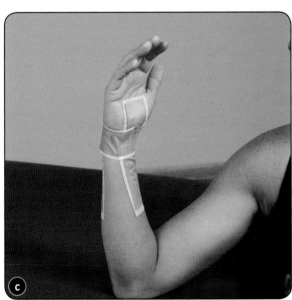

WRIST FLEXION
OR EXTENSION BLOCK

Indications

An extension block limits active wrist extension and is effective for treating pronator syndrome or pain at the anterior elbow with wrist flexion and elbow extension; a flexor block limits active wrist flexion.

Client's Position

The client is sitting with the arm on a table.

Physical Therapist's Position

The PT is sitting at the table, opposite the client.

Application Guidelines

1. For an extension block, apply underwrap with the wrist in a neutral position, placing one strip from the volar midforearm to 1 inch (2.5 cm) distal to the radial styloid process on the palmar hand.

2. Follow with strapping tape (*a*).

3. For a flexion block, apply underwrap and strapping tape from the dorsal midforearm to 1 inch (2.5 cm) distal to the radial styloid process (*b*).

4. For either application, pull distally during application and finish with an anchor strip on underwrap and strapping tape around the wrist.

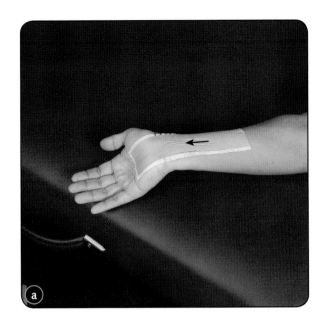 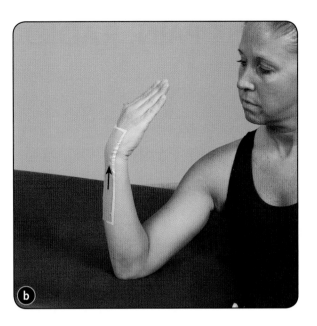

WRIST PAIN, RADIOCARPAL GLIDE

Indications

This technique is effective for treating pain at the wrist with flexion or extension.

Client's Position

The client is sitting with the elbow on a table or is supine with the elbow flexed.

Physical Therapist's Position

The PT is facing the client's hand. A second clinician is required to assist with taping.

Screen

Perform the radiocarpal accessory motion test (Mulligan 1999). At the ulnar styloid, apply a radial glide with your web space to the proximal carpals while stabilizing the radius with the other hand (*a*).

Application Guidelines (Mulligan)

1. Use half width of strapping tape. One clinician maintains the radiocarpal glide while a second clinician applies underwrap then strapping tape to the palmar wrist distal to the ulnar styloid and around the dorsal wrist while gliding; anchor to the tape at the starting point (*b-d*).

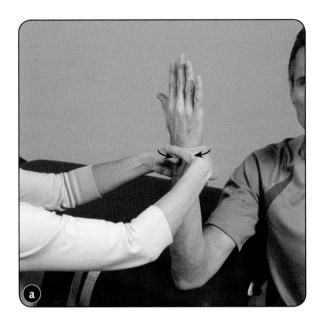

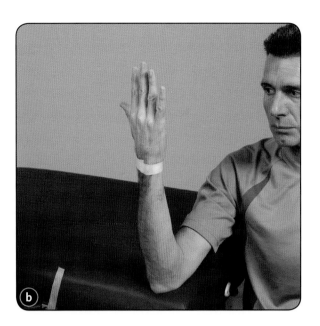

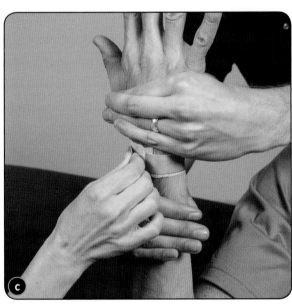

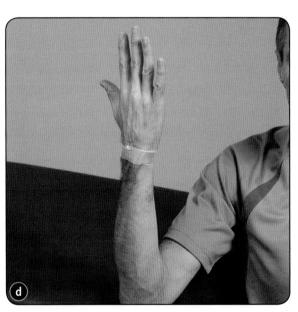

FIFTH METACARPAL
DORSAL GLIDE

Indications

This technique is effective for treating pain at the lateral fourth and fifth metacarpals or at the ulnar wrist with gripping.

Client's Position

The client is sitting with the arm on a table, palm down.

Physical Therapist's Position

The PT is sitting at the table, opposite the client. A second clinician is required to assist with taping.

Screen

Perform an accessory motion test of the dorsal fifth metacarpal (with pain at the fourth or fifth metacarpal when gripping) (a). If pain is diminished when a dorsal glide to the fifth metacarpal is done, this technique would be helpful.

Application Guidelines (Mulligan)

1. Apply an upward (dorsal) glide on the fifth metacarpal while stabilizing the fourth metacarpal.
2. Apply underwrap, starting at the palmar fifth metacarpal (b).
3. Follow with half-width strapping tape, maintaining force dorsally and radially (c); anchor on the medial forearm (d-e).

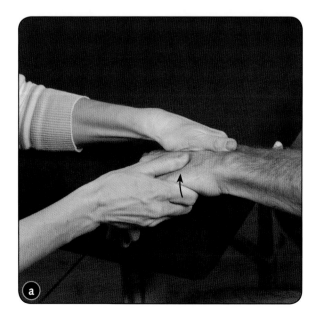

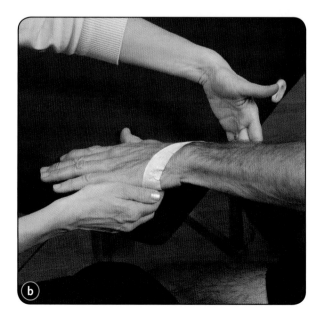

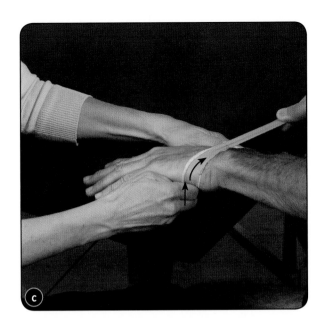

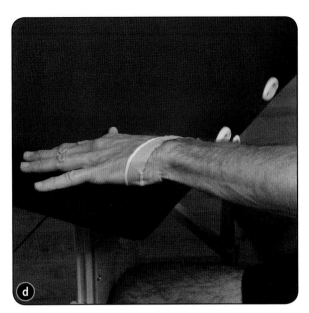

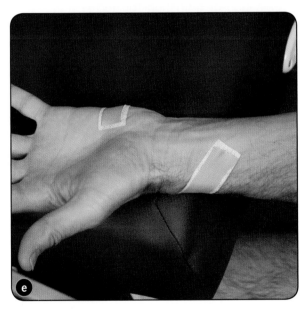

VENTRAL ULNAR GLIDE

Indications

This technique is effective for treating pain at the distal radioulnar joint with supination or pronation.

Client's Position

The client is standing with the arm at the side.

Physical Therapist's Position

The PT is standing, facing the affected arm. A second clinician is required to assist with taping.

Screen

Apply a ventral glide to the distal ulna during supination or pronation for decrease in symptoms (*a*) (Mulligan 1999).

Application Guidelines (Mulligan)

1. Palpate the distal ulna, and apply a palmar glide with supination.
2. The second clinician applies underwrap on the volar wrist, not wrapping around the wrist completely (*b*).
3. Follow with half-width strapping tape, maintaining pressure while pulling the tape palmarly and anchoring it on the radius. The tape should not completely wrap around the wrist (*c-d*).

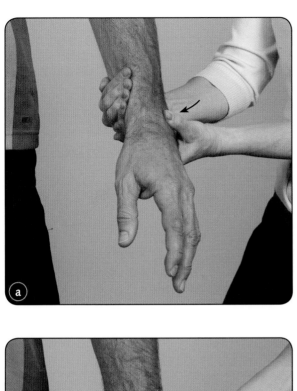

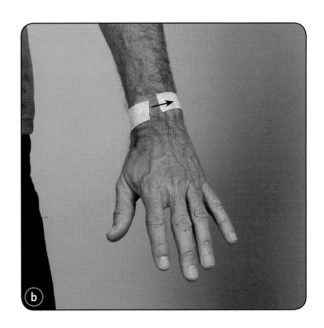

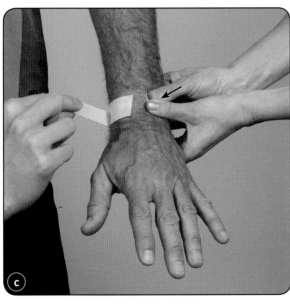

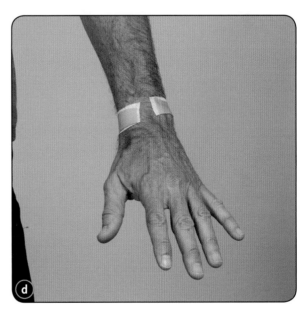

TRAPEZIUM GLIDE

Indication

This technique is effective for treating pain at the first metacarpal joint and trapezium with thumb extension.

Client's Position

The client is sitting at a table or is standing.

Physical Therapist's Position

The PT is sitting, using one hand to grip the client's wrist and thumb at the anatomical snuffbox and the other hand to stabilize the carpals. A second clinician is required to assist with taping.

Screen

Perform the trapezium accessory movement test for wrist pain (a) (Mulligan 1999). Stabilize the first metacapal and apply an anterolateral glide to the trapezium with thumb extension. If this decreases symptoms, apply the technique.

Application Guidelines (Mulligan)

1. One clinician maintains the screening position described above.
2. The second clinician applies underwrap palmarly around the base of the thumb to the ulna (b).
3. Follow with half-width strapping tape, anchoring to the ulna (c-d).

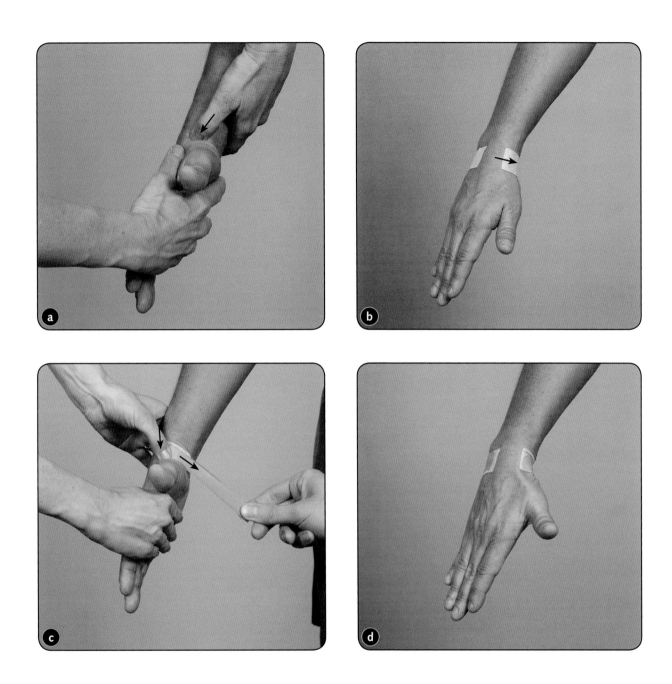

THUMB BLOCK

Indications

This technique is effective for treating De Quervain's tenosynovitis, UCL tears or instability, gamekeeper's thumb, and skier's thumb.

Client's Position

The client is sitting with the arm on a table.

Physical Therapist's Position

The PT is sitting at the table, opposite the client.

Application Guidelines

1. Apply underwrap (width may need to be cut in half depending on hand size), starting at the snuffbox and moving up through the web space of the thumb and first finger and around the thumb toward the ulnar volar wrist (a).

2. Apply strapping tape in the same manner following the underwrap (b-d).

3. If necessary, apply a strip of underwrap and strapping tape around the wrist to discourage ulnar deviation (e-f).

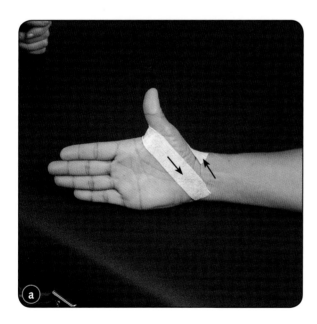

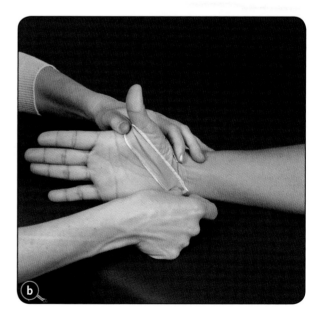

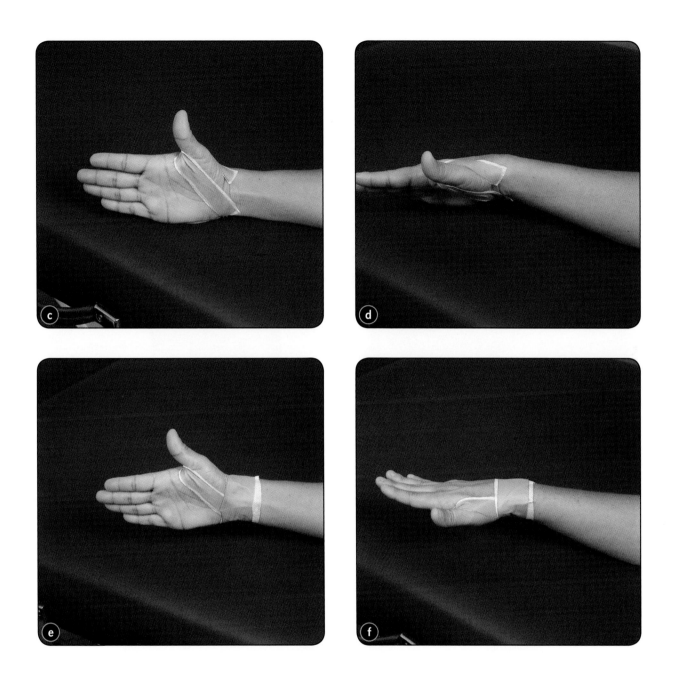

BRACES

The following braces simulate taping techniques (for use when continuous support is not necessary, during activity only):

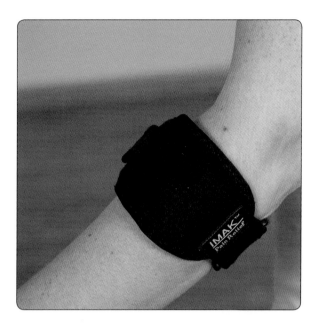

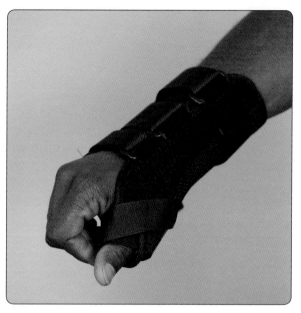

Epicondylitis strap: Available over the counter, this strap is worn distal to the elbow (when nerve compression has been ruled out) to treat lateral or medial epicondylitis. A neutral wrist splint may also be beneficial at night for epicondylitis.

Hand- or wrist-based thumb spica splints: Medical supply stores carry these splints that stabilize the thumb for treatment of De Quervain's tenosynovitis, UCL tears or instability, gamekeeper's thumb, and skier's thumb; however, sometimes a custom splint is indicated, so it is best to consult a hand therapist (PT or OT) first.

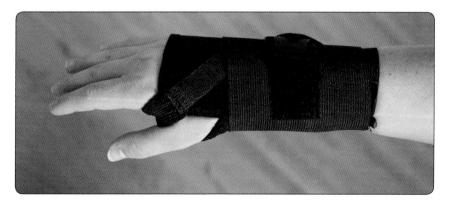

Neutral wrist splint: Available over the counter or sometimes custom made, this type of splint is used primarily at night to treat carpal tunnel syndrome, but it can be used during the day for activities involving excessive use of the hand and wrist.

CASE STUDIES

Taping and lateral epicondylitis (tennis elbow).

A 35-year-old female lifted with too wide a grip a heavy 5-inch (13 cm) wide box and complained of lateral epicondyle pain with resistance to gripping. Tests for nerve entrapment about the lateral elbow were negative. Treatment included soft tissue mobilization to the lateral extensor mass, radial head mobilization with movement (MWM), iontophoresis, and eccentric wrist extension strengthening. Her symptoms were easily exacerbated at her job as a massage therapist. She could not use a tennis elbow brace at work because of its bulk. Epicondylitis strapping was applied before her workday, and she reported less pain. Her symptoms were completely resolved in 1 month without missing work (she was unable financially to take time off work to rest the arm as recommended).

Taping and medial epicondylitis (golfer's elbow).

A 47-year-old male was doing heavy landscaping one weekend and experienced bilateral forearm and elbow pain. The following weekend he played 18 holes of golf and afterward had constant soreness of the medial epicondyle on one arm. The soreness persisted, and he was unable to tolerate practicing at the driving range. He had pain with resisted grip and wrist flexion and tenderness over the medial epicondyle. The patient was treated in physical therapy with soft tissue mobilization, stretching, and pain-free strengthening. He was taped with forearm strapping and was able to go to the driving range with only mild pain while taped. He was advised to wear a forearm strap brace only during heavy activities such as golfing and yard work. Trigger point dry needling treatment was continued in the clinic once weekly until symptoms were completely resolved, and he was doing all his usual activities brace free in 2 months.

REFERENCES

Ackermann, B., R. Adams, and E. Marshall. 2002. The effect of scapula taping on electromyographic activity and musical performance in professional violinists. *Australian Journal of Physiotherapy* 48 (3): 197-203.

Adamczyk, A., W. Kiebzak, M. Wilk-Franczuk, and Z. Sliwinski. 2009. Effectiveness of holistic physiotherapy for low back pain. *Ortopedia, Traumatologia, Rehabilitacja* 11:562.

Adams, E., and C. Madden. 2009. Cuboid subluxation: A case study and review of the literature. *Current Sports Medicine Reports* 8:300.

Alexander, C., S. Stynes, A. Thomas, J. Lewis, and P. Harrison. 2003. Does tape facilitate or inhibit the lower fibres of trapezius? *Manual Therapy* 8 (1): 37-41.

Alt, W., H. Lohrer, and A. Gollhofer. 1999. Functional properties of adhesive ankle taping: Neuromuscular and mechanical effects before and after exercise. *Foot and Ankle International* 4:238-245.

Ancliffe, J. 1992. Strapping the shoulder in patients following a cerebrovascular accident (CVA): A pilot study. *Australian Journal of Physiotherapy* 38:37-41.

Aspegren, D., T. Hyde, and M. Miller. 2007. Conservative treatment of a female collegiate volleyball player with costochondritis. *Journal of Manipulative and Physiological Therapeutics* 30 (4): 321-325.

Ator, R., K. Gunn, T. McPoil, and H. Knecht. 1991. The effect of adhesive strapping on medial longitudinal arch support before and after exercise. *Journal of Orthopedic and Sports Physical Therapy* 14 (1): 18-23.

Bennell, K., S. Coburn, E. Wee, S. Green, A. Harris, A. Forbes, and R. Buchbinder. 2007. Efficacy and cost-effectiveness of a physiotherapy program for chronic rotator cuff pathology: A protocol for a randomised, double-blind, placebo-controlled trial. *BMC Musculoskeletal Disorders* 8 (August 31): 86.

Beumer, A., Swierstra B., and P Mulder. 2002. Clinical diagnosis of syndesmotic ankle instability: evaluation of stress tests behind the curtain. *Acta Orthop Scand.* 73: 667-9.

Bhave, A., D. Paley, and J. Herzenberg. 1999. Improvement in gait parameters after lengthening for the treatment of limb-length discrepancy. *Journal of Bone and Joint Surgery (American)* 81:529-534.

Blustein, S., and J. D'Amico. 1985. Limb length discrepancy: Identification, clinical significance, and management. *Journal of the American Podiatric Medical Association* 75 (4): 200-206.

Bockrath, K., C. Wooden, T. Worrell, C. Ingersoll, and J. Farr. 1993. Effects of patella taping on patella position and perceived pain. *Medicine and Science in Sports and Exercise* 25:989-992.

Borkholder, C., V. Hill, and E. Fess. 2004. The efficacy of splinting for lateral epicondylitis: A systematic review. *Journal of Hand Therapy* 17:181-199.

Bragg, R., J. MacMahon, E. Overom, S. Yerby, G. Matheson, D. Carter, and P. Andriacchi. 2002. Failure and fatigue characteristics of adhesive athletic tape. *Medicine and Science in Sports and Exercise* 33 (3): 403-410.

Brown, G., R. Donatelli, P. Catlin, and M. Wooden. 1995. The effect of two types of foot orthoses on rearfoot mechanics. *Journal of Orthopedic and Sports Physical Therapy* 21 (5): 258-267.

Butlers, K., and K. Singer. 1994. Nerve lesions of the arm and elbow. In *Orthopedic Sports Medicine: Principles and Practice.* Philadelphia: Saunders.

Callaghan, M.J., J. Selfe, A. McHenry, and J. Oldham. 2008. Effects of patellar taping on knee joint proprioception in patients with patellofemoral pain syndrome. *Manual Therapy* 13 (3): 192-199.

Carda, S., and F. Molteni. 2005. Taping versus electrical stimulation after botulinum toxin type A injection for wrist and finger spasticity: A case-control study. *Clinical Rehabilitation* 19 (6): 621-626.

Carter, K., and N. Chockalingam. 2009. An assessment of strapping techniques commonly used for pronated foot deformities. *Journal of the American Podiatric Medical Association* 99 (5): 391-398.

Cerny, K. 1995. Vastus medialis oblique/vastus lateralis muscle activity ratios for selected exercises in persons with and without patellofemoral pain syndrome. *Physical Therapy* 75:672-683.

Christou, E. 2004. Patellar taping increases vastus medialis oblique activity in the presence of patellofemoral pain. *Journal of Electromyography and Kinesiology* 14:495-504.

Cleland, J. 2007. *Orthopedic Clinical Exam: An Evidence Based Approach for Physical Therapists*. Philadelphia: Saunders.

Conway, A., T. Malone, and P. Conway. 1992. Patellar alignment/tracking alteration: Effect on force output and perceived pain. *Isokinetics and Exercise Science* 2:9-17.

Cools, A., E. Witvrouw, L. Danneels, and D. Cambier. 2002. Does taping influence electromyographic muscle activity in the scapular rotators in healthy shoulders? *Manual Therapy* 7 (3): 154-162.

Cowan, S., K. Bennell, K. Crossley, P. Hodges, and J. McConnell. 2002. Physiotherapy treatment changes EMG onset timing of VMO relative to VL in subjects with patellofemoral pain syndrome: A randomised, double-blind, placebo-controlled trial. *Medicine and Science in Sports and Exercise* 34 (12): 1879-1885.

Crossley, K., K. Bennell, S. Green, S. Cowan, and J. McConnell. 2002. Physical therapy for patellofemoral pain: A randomized, double-blinded, placebo-controlled trial. *American Journal of Sports Medicine* 30 (6): 857-865.

Crossley, K., K. Bennell, S. Green, and J. McConnell. 2001. A systematic review of physical interventions for patellofemoral pain syndrome. *Clinical Journal of Sports Medicine* 11 (2): 103.

Crossley, K., S. Cowan, K. Bennell, and J. McConnell. 2000. Patellar taping: Is clinical success supported by scientific evidence? *Manual Therapy* 5 (3): 142-150.

Crossley, K., G. Marino, M. Macilquham, A. Schache, and R. Hinman. 2009. Can patellar tape reduce the patellar malalignment and pain associated with patellofemoral osteoarthritis? *Arthritis and Rheumatism* 61:1719.

Crowell, R., and J. Paolino. 2005. *Mulligan Taping Techniques*. DVD. East Hampstead, NH: Northeast Seminars.

Cushnaghan, J., C. McCarthy, and P. Dieppe. 1994. Taping the patella medially: A new treatment for osteoarthritis of the knee joint? *British Medical Journal* 308:753-755.

D'Amico, J., H. Dinowitz, and M. Polchaninoff. 1985. Limb length discrepancy: An electromyographic analysis. *Journal of the American Podiatric Medical Association* 75 (12): 639-643.

Defrin, R., S. Benyamin, R. Aldubi, C. Pick. 2005. Conservative correction of leg-length discrepancies of 10 mm or less for relief of chronic low back pain. *Archives of Physical Medicine and Rehabilitation* 86:2075-2080.

Delahunt, E., A. McGrath, N. Doran, and G. Coughlan. 2010. Effect of taping on actual and perceived dynamic postural stability in persons with chronic ankle instability. *Archives of Physical Medicine and Rehabilitation* 91 (9): 1383-1389.

Delahunt, E., J. O'Driscoll, and K. Moran. 2009. Effects of taping and exercise on ankle joint movement in subjects with chronic ankle instability: A preliminary investigation. *Archives of Physical Medicine and Rehabilitation* 90:1418.

Derasari, A., T. Brindle, K. Alter, and F. Sheehan. 2010. McConnell taping shifts the patella inferiorly in patients with patellofemoral pain: A dynamic magnetic resonance imaging study. *Physical Therapy* 90 (3): 411.

Eckstrom, R., and K. Holden. 2002. Examination of and intervention for patients with chronic lateral elbow pain with signs of nerve entrapment. *Physical Therapy* 82:1077-1086.

Ernst, G., J. Kawaguchi, and E. Saliba. 1999. Effect of patellar taping on knee kinetics of patients with patellofemoral pain syndrome. *Journal of Orthopedic and Sports Physical Therapy* 29: 661-667.

Farrell, E., E. Naber, and P. Geigle. 2010. Description of a multifaceted rehabilitation program including overground gait training for a child with cerebral palsy: A case report. *Physiotherapy Theory and Practice* 26 (1): 56-61.

Fitzgerald, G., and P. McClure. 1995. Reliability of measurements obtained with four tests for patellofemoral alignment. *Physical Therapy* 75:84-92.

Franettovich, M., A. Chapman, P. Blanch, and B. Vicenzino. 2008. A physiological and psychological basis for anti-pronation taping from a critical review of the literature. *Sports Medicine* 38 (8): 617-631.

Franettovich, M., A. Chapman, P. Blanch, and B. Vicenzino. 2009. Continual use of augmented low-Dye taping increases arch height in standing but does not influence neuromotor control of gait. *Gait and Posture* 31 (2): 247-250.

Friberg, O., M. Nurminen, K. Korhonen, E. Soininen, and T. Manttari. 1983. Accuracy and precision of clinical estimation of leg length inequality and lumbar scoliosis: Comparison of clinical and radiological measurements. *International Disability Studies* 10 (2): 49-53.

Fu, T., A. Wong, Y. Pei, K. Wu, S. Chou, and Y. Lin. 2008. Effect of Kinesio taping on muscle strength in athletes: A pilot study. *Journal of Science and Medicine in Sport* 11 (2): 198-201.

García-Muro, F., A. Rodríguez-Fernández, and A. Herrero-de-Lucas. 2010. Treatment of myofascial pain in the shoulder with Kinesio taping: A case report. *Manual Therapy* 15 (3): 292-295.

Genova, J., and M. Gross. 2000. Effect of foot orthotics on calcaneal eversion during standing and treadmill walking for subjects with abnormal pronation. *Journal of Orthopedic and Sports Physical Therapy* 30 (11): 664-675.

Giles, L.G., and J. Taylor. 1981. Low-back pain associated with leg length inequality. *Spine* 6 (5): 510-521.

Gilleard, W., J. McConnell, and D. Parsons. 1998. The effect of patellar taping on the onset of vastus medialis obliquus and vastus lateralis muscle activity in persons with patellofemoral pain. *Physical Therapy* 78:25-31.

González-Iglesias, J., C. Fernández-de-Las-Peñas, J.A. Cleland, P. Huijbregts, and M. Del Rosario Gutiérrez-Vega. 2009. Short-term effects of cervical Kinesio taping on pain and cervical range of motion in patients with acute whiplash injury: A randomized clinical trial. *Journal of Orthopedic and Sports Physical Therapy* 39 (7): 515-521.

Greig, M., K. Bennell, A. Briggs, and P. Hodges. 2008. Postural taping decreases thoracic kyphosis but does not influence trunk muscle electromyographic activity or balance in women with osteoporosis. *Manual Therapy* 13 (3): 249-257.

Grelsamer, R.P., and J. McConnell. 1998. *The Patella: A Team Approach.* Gaithersburg, MD: Aspen.

Griffin, A., and J. Bernhardt. 2006. Strapping the hemiplegic shoulder prevents development of pain during rehabilitation: A randomized controlled trial. *Clinical Rehabilitation* 20 (4): 287-295.

Gross, M. Limb length inequality: Clinical implications for assessment and intervention. *Journal of Orthopedic and Sports Physical Therapy* 33:221-234.

Gross, M. 1995. Lower quarter screening for skeletal malalignment: Suggestions for orthotics and shoewear. *Journal of Orthopedic and Sports Physical Therapy* 21:389-405.

Gross, R. 1983. Leg length discrepancy in marathon runners. *American Journal of Sports Medicine* 11 (3): 121-124.

Hadala, M., and C. Barrios. 2009. Different strategies for sports injury prevention in an America's Cup yachting crew. *Medicine and Science in Sports and Exercise* 41 (8): 1587-1596.

Hall, M., W. Ferrell, R. Sturrock, D. Hamblen and R. Baxendale. 1995. The effect of the hypermobility syndrome on knee joint proprioception, *British Journal of Rheumatology* 34: 121–125.

Herrington, L. 2001. The effect of patellar taping on quadriceps peak torque and perceived pain: A preliminary study. *Physical Therapy in Sport* 2 (1): 23-28.

Herrington, L. 2004. The effect of patella taping on quadriceps strength and functional performance in normal subjects. *Physical Therapy in Sport* 5 (1): 33-36.

Herrington, L. 2010. The effect of patellar taping on patellar position measured using ultrasound scanning. *Knee* 17 (2): 132-134.

Herrington, L., and S. Al-Shebli. 2006. Effect of ankle taping on vertical jump in male volleyball players before and after exercise. *Physical Therapy in Sport* 7 (4): 175-176.

Herrington, L., and C. Payton. 1997. Effect of corrective taping of the patella on patients with patellofemoral pain. *Physiotherapy* 83:566-572.

Hertling, D., and R. Kessler. 1996. *Management of Common Musculoskeletal Disorders*, 3rd ed. Philadelphia: Lippincott Williams & Wilkins.

Hinman, R., K. Crossley, J. McConnell, and K. Bennell. 2003. Efficacy of knee tape in the management of osteoarthritis of the knee: Blinded randomized controlled trial. *British Medical Journal* 327:135.

Hopper, D., K. Samsson, T. Hulenik, C. Ng, T. Hall, and K. Robinson. 2009. The influence of Mulligan ankle taping during balance performance in subjects with unilateral chronic ankle instability. *Physical Therapy in Sport* 10 (4): 125-130.

Host, H. 1995. Scapular taping in the treatment of anterior shoulder impingement. *Physical Therapy* 75 (9): 803-812.

Hsu, Y., W. Chen, H. Lin, W. Wang, and Y. Shih. 2009. The effects of taping on scapular kinematics and muscle performance in baseball players with shoulder impingement syndrome. *Journal of Electromyography and Kinesiology* 19 (6): 1092-1099.

Hughes, T., and P. Rochester. 2008. The effects of proprioceptive exercises and taping on proprioception in subjects with functional ankle instability: A review of literature. *Physical Therapy in Sport* 9:136-147.

Hyland, M.R., A. Webber-Gaffney, L. Cohen, and P. Lichtman. 2006. Randomized controlled trial of calcaneal taping, sham taping, and plantar fascia stretching for the short-term management of plantar heel pain. *Journal of Orthopedic and Sports Physical Therapy* 36:364-371.

Iosa, M., D. Morelli, M.V. Nanni, C. Veredice, T. Marro, A. Medici, S. Paolucci, and C. Mazza. 2010. Functional taping: A promising technique for children with cerebral palsy. *Developmental Medicine and Child Neurology* 52 (6): 587-589.

Jaraczewska, E., and C. Long. 2006. Kinesio taping in stroke: Improving functional use of the upper extremity in hemiplegia. *Topics in Stroke Rehabilitation* 13 (3): 31-42.

Kaufman, K., L. Miller, and D. Sutherland. 1996. Gait asymmetry in patients with limb length inequality. *Journal of Pediatric Orthopedics* 16:144-150.

Kendall H., and F. Kendall. 1999. *Muscles: Testing and Function*. Baltimore: William & Wilkins.

Kilbreath, S., S. Perkins, J. Crosbie, and J. McConnell. 2006. Gluteal taping improves hip extension during stance phase of walking following stroke. *Australian Journal of Physiotherapy* 52 (1): 53-56.

Lampe, H.I., B. Swierstra, and A. Diepstraten. 1996. Measurement of limb length inequality: Comparison of clinical methods with orthoradiography in 190 children. *Acta Orthopaedica Scandinavica* 67 (3): 242-244.

Lange, B., L. Chipchase, and A. Evans. 2004. An assessment of strapping techniques commonly used for pronated foot deformities: The effect of low-Dye taping on plantar pressures, during gait, in subjects with navicular drop exceeding 10 mm. *Journal of Orthopedic and Sports Physical Therapy* 34:201-209.

Lewis, J.S., C. Wright, and A. Green. 2005. Subacromial impingement syndrome: The effect of changing posture on shoulder range of movement. *Journal of Orthopedic and Sports Physical Therapy* 35 (2): 72-87.

Lo, I., B. Nonweiler, M. Woolfrey, R Litchfield, A Kirkley. 2004. An evaluation of apprehension, relocation, and surprise tests for anterior shoulder instability. *American Journal of Sports Medicine* 32:301-307.

Magee, D.J. 2006. *Orthopedic Physical Assessment*, 4th ed. St Louis: Saunders Elsevier.

Maguire, C., J. Sieben, M. Frank, and J. Romkes. 2010. Hip abductor control in walking following stroke: The immediate effect of canes, taping and TheraTogs on gait. *Clinical Rehabilitation* 24 (1): 37-45.

McConnell J., 1986. The management of chondromalacia patellae: a long-term solution. *Australian Journal of Physiother*apy 32: 215–33.

McConnell, J. 2000. A novel approach to pain relief pre therapeutic exercise. *Journal of Science and Medicine in Sport* 3:325-334.

McConnell, J. 2002. Recalcitrant chronic low back and leg pain: A new theory and different approach to management. *Manual Therapy* 7 (4): 183-192.

McConnell, J. 2010. McConnell Approach to the Lower Extremity. Course notes.

McPoil, T. 1988. Footwear. *Physical Therapy* 68 (12): 1857-1865.

McPoil, T.G., and M. Cornwall. 2000. The effect of foot orthoses on transverse tibial rotation during walking. *Journal of the American Podiatric Medical Association* 90 (1): 2-11.

McPoil, T.G., and M. Cornwall. 2007. Foot and Ankle Update: Biomechanics, Evaluation, and Orthotic Intervention. Course notes, APTA Annual Conference, Denver, CO.

Meier, K., T. McPoil, M. Cornwall, and T. Lyle. 2008. Use of antipronation taping to determine foot orthoses prescription: A case series. *Research in Sports Medicine* 16 (4): 257-271.

Miller, P., and P. Osmotherly. 2009. Does scapula taping facilitate recovery for shoulder impingement symptoms? A pilot randomized controlled trial. *Journal of Manual and Manipulative Therapy* 17:E6.

Moiler, K., T. Hall, and K. Robinson. 2006. The role of fibular tape in the prevention of ankle injury in basketball: A pilot study. *Journal of Orthopedic and Sports Physical Therapy* 36 (9): 661-668.

Morin, L., and G. Bravo. 1997. Strapping the hemiplegic shoulder: A radiographic evaluation of its efficacy to reduce subluxation. *Physiotherapy Canada* (Spring): 103-108.

Mulligan, B.R. 1999. *Manual Therapy: 'NAGS', 'SNAGS', and 'MWMS' etc.* Wellington, NZ: Plane View Services.

Ng, G., and J. Cheng 2002. The effects of patellar taping on pain and neuromuscular performance in subjects with patellofemoral pain syndrome. *Clinical Rehabilitation* 16:821-827.

Ng, G.Y, and P. Wong. 2009. Patellar taping affects vastus medialis obliquus activation in subjects with patellofemoral pain before and after quadriceps muscle fatigue. *Clinical Rehabilitation* 23 (8): 705-713.

Nolan, D., N. Kennedy, K. Moiler, T. Hall, and K. Robinson. 2009. Effects of low-Dye taping on plantar pressure pre and post exercise: An exploratory study. *BMC Musculoskeletal Disorders* 10 (Apr 21): 40.

Osborne, H., and G. Allison. 2006. Treatment of plantar fasciitis by low-Dye taping and iontophoresis: Short term results of a double blinded, randomized, placebo controlled clinical trial of dexamethasone and acetic acid. *British Journal of Sports Medicine* (February): 1-5.

Papaioannou, T., I. Stokes, and J. Kenwright. 1982. Scoliosis associated with limb-length inequality. *Journal of Bone and Joint Surgery (American)* 64 (1): 59-62.

Passerallo, A., and G. Calabrese. 1994. Improving traditional ankle taping techniques with rigid strapping tape. *Journal of Athletic Training* 29 (1): 76-77.

Pecina, M., J. Krmpotic-Nemanic, and A. Markiewitz. 1991. *Tunnel Syndromes*. Boca Raton, FL: CRC Press.

Perrin, D. 2005. *Athletic Taping and Bracing*, 2nd ed. Champaign, IL: Human Kinetics.

Peterson, C. 2004. The use of electrical stimulation and taping to address shoulder subluxation for a patient with central cord syndrome. *Physical Therapy* 84 (7): 634-643.

Plancher, K.D., R.K. Peterson, and J.B. Steichen. 1996. Compressive neuropathies and tendinopathies in the athletic elbow and wrist. *Clinics in Sports Medicine* 15:331-372.

Powers, C., R. Landel, T. Sosnick, J. Kirby, K. Mengel, A. Cheney, and J. Perry. 1997. The effects of patellar taping on stride characteristics and joint motion in subjects with patellofemoral pain. *Journal of Orthopedic and Sports Physical Therapy* 26:286-291.

Prost, A. 1990. Place de la kinesitherapie dans le traitement du syndrome de la traversee thoraco-brachiale. *Kinesitherapie Scientifique* 288: 5-22.

Revel, M., B. Amor. 1983. Rehabilitation of cervico-thoraco-brachial outlet syndrome. *Phlebologie* 36: 157-65.

Quilty, B., M. Tucker, R. Campbell, and P. Dieppe. 2003. Physiotherapy, including quadriceps exercises and patellar taping, for knee osteoarthritis with predominant patello-femoral joint involvement: Randomized controlled trial. *Journal of Rheumatology* 30:1311-1317.

Richmond, J., D. Hunter, J. Irrgang, M.H. Jones, B. Levy, R. Marx, L. Snyder-Mackler, W.C. Watters 3rd, R.H. Haralson 3rd, C.M. Turkelson, J.L. Wies, K.M. Boyer, S. Anderson, J. St Andre, P. Sluka, R. McGowan, and American Academy of Orthopaedic Surgeons. 2009. Treatment of osteoarthritis of the knee (nonarthroplasty). *Journal of the American Academy of Orthopedic Surgeons* 17 (9): 591-600.

Russo, S.J., and L. Chipchase. 2001. The effect of low-Dye taping on peak plantar pressures of normal feet during gait. *Australian Journal of Physiotherapy* 47 (4): 239-244.

Schoffl, I., F. Einwag, W. Strecker, F. Hennig, and V. Schoffl. 2007. Impact of taping after finger flexor tendon pulley ruptures in rock climbers. *Journal of Applied Biomechanics* 23 (1): 52-62.

Selkowitz, D.M., C. Chaney, S. Stuckey, and G. Vlad. 2007. The effects of scapular taping on the surface electromyographic signal amplitude of shoulder girdle muscles during upper extremity elevation in individuals with suspected shoulder impingement syndrome. *Journal of Orthopedic and Sports Physical Therapy* 37 (11): 694-702.

Shamus, J., and E. Shamus. 1997. A taping technique for the treatment of acromioclavicular joint sprains: A case study. *Journal of Orthopedic and Sports Physical Therapy* 25:390-394.

Simmonds, J.V., and R. Keer. 2007. Hypermobility and the hypermobility syndrome. *Manual Therapy* 12 (4): 298-309.

Smith, M., V. Sparkes, M. Busse, and S. Enright. 2009. Upper and lower trapezius muscle activity in subjects with subacromial impingement symptoms: Is there imbalance and can taping change it? *Physical Therapy in Sport* 10 (2): 45-50.

Sparkes, V. 2006. The immediate effect of scapular taping on surface electromyographic activity of the scapular rotators in swimmers with subacromial impingement symptoms. *Physical Therapy in Sport* 7:4-17.

Stoffel, K., R. Nicholls, A. Winata, A. Dempsey, J. Boyle, and D. Lloyd. 2010. The effect of ankle taping on knee and ankle joint biomechanics in sporting tasks. *Medicine and Science in Sports and Exercise* 42 (11): 2089-2097.

Subotnick, S. 1981. Limb length discrepancies of the lower extremity (the short leg syndrome). *Journal of Orthopedic and Sports Physical Therapy* 3:11-16.

Thelen, M.D., Dauber J.A, and P. Stoneman. 2008. The clinical efficacy of Kinesio tape for shoulder pain: A randomized, double-blinded, clinical trial. *Journal of Orthopedic and Sports Physical Therapy* 38 (7): 389-395.

Tobin, S., and G. Robinson. 2000. The effect of McConnell's vastusl lateralis inhibition taping technique on vastus lateralis and vastus medialis obliquus activity. *Physiotherapy* 86: 173-183. Van de Water, A., and C. Speksnijder. 2010. Efficacy of taping for the treatment of plantar fasciosis: A systematic review of controlled trials. *Journal of the American Podiatric Medical Association* 100:41-51.

Vanti, C., L. Natalini, A. Romeo, D. Tosarelli, and P. Pillastrini. 2007. Conservative treatment of thoracic outlet syndrome: A review of the literature. *Europa Medicophysica* 43 (1): 55-70.

Vicenzino, B. 2003. Lateral epicondylalgia: A musculoskeletal physiotherapy perspective. *Manual Therapy* 8 (2): 66-79.

Vicenzino, B. 2004. Foot orthotics in the treatment of lower limb conditions: A musculoskeletal physiotherapy perspective. *Manual Therapy* 9 (4): 185-196.

Vicenzino, B., J. Brooksbank, J. Minto, S. Offord, and A. Paungmali. 2003. Initial effects of elbow taping on pain-free grip strength and pressure pain threshold. *Journal of Orthopedic and Sports Physical Therapy* 33 (7): 400-407.

Vicenzino, B., T. McPoil, and S. Buckland. 2007. Plantar foot pressures after the augmented low Dye taping technique. *Journal of Athletic Training* 42 (3): 374-380.

Vicenzino, B., A. Paungmali, and P. Teys. 2007. Mulligan's mobilization with movement, positional faults and pain relief: Current concepts from a critical review of literature. *Manual Therapy* 12:98-108.

Warden, S.J., R. Hinman, M. Watson Jr., K. Avin, A. Bialocerkowski, and K. Crossley. 2008. Patellar taping and bracing for the treatment of chronic knee pain: A systematic review and meta-analysis. *Arthritis and Rheumatism* 59:73-83.

Whittingham, M., S. Palmer, and F. MacMillan. 2004. Effects of taping on pain and function in patellofemoral pain syndrome: A randomized controlled trial. *Journal of Orthopedic and Sports Physical Therapy* 34 (9): 504-510.

Wilson, T., N. Carter, and G. Thomas. 2003. A multicenter, single-masked study of medial, neutral, and lateral patellar taping in individuals with patellofemoral pain syndrome. *Journal of Orthopedic and Sports Physical Therapy* 33:437-443.

Yasukawa, A., P. Patel, and C. Sisung. 2006. Pilot study: Investigating the effects of Kinesio taping in an acute pediatric rehabilitation setting. *American Journal of Occupational Therapy* 60 (1): 104-110.

ABOUT THE AUTHOR

Anne Keil, PT, DPT, is a physical therapist and supervisor of rehabilitation services at the University of Colorado Hospital at Stapleton and Park Meadows Rehabilitation Clinics in Denver. Dr. Keil has worked in a variety of areas, including outpatient orthopedics, neurology, inpatient, skilled nursing, rehabilitation, and home health care. Working in facilities or countries that did not have many physical therapy resources, Dr. Keil became interested in taping as a low-cost adjunct to treatment and an effective alternative to bracing.

Dr. Keil received her doctorate in physical therapy in 2005 from Simmons College in Boston, Massachusetts. She earned her BS in physical therapy in 1991 and BS in community health science in 1989 from California State University at Fresno. Dr. Keil is a member of the American Physical Therapy Association (APTA).

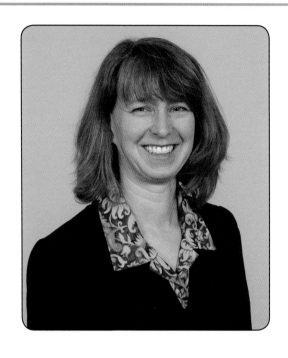

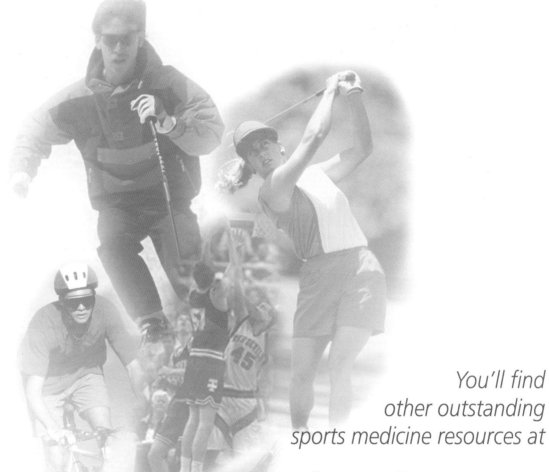